More Praise for *100 Questions & Answers About Psoriasis, Second Edition*

"[If] you are a person who is educated and informed about psoriasis, you will be more satisfied with your treatment and your doctor, and will have greater confidence in your future. We are grateful to Drs. Alexa Kimball and Kendra Bergstrom for helping to generate awareness and understanding about this chronic, lifelong disease."

Gail Zimmerman

Former President and CEO, National Psoriasis Foundation

"Psoriasis is a common skin disease that affects millions of people around the world. In recent years, a revolution has occurred in treatment options available for psoriasis. Drs. Bergstrom and Kimball have given us a clearly written guide to help psoriasis patients understand these options and select the appropriate treatment for this life-crippling disease."

Fred F. Castrow II, MD

Past President, American Academy of Dermatology

100 Questions & Answers About Psoriasis
Second Edition

Kendra Gail Bergstrom, MD
Pacific Medical Centers
Seattle, Washington

Alexa Boer Kimball, MD, MPH
Vice Chair, Department of Dermatology
Massachusetts General Hospital
Boston, Massachusetts

JONES AND BARTLETT PUBLISHERS
Sudbury, Massachusetts
BOSTON   TORONTO   LONDON   SINGAPORE

World Headquarters

Jones and Bartlett Publishers
40 Tall Pine Drive
Sudbury, MA 01776
978-443-5000
info@jbpub.com
www.jbpub.com

Jones and Bartlett Publishers
Canada
6339 Ormindale Way
Mississauga, Ontario L5V 1J2
Canada

Jones and Bartlett Publishers
International
Barb House, Barb Mews
London W6 7PA
United Kingdom

Jones and Bartlett's books and products are available through most bookstores and online book-sellers. To contact Jones and Bartlett Publishers directly, call 800-832-0034, fax 978-443-8000, or visit our website, www.jbpub.com.

Substantial discounts on bulk quantities of Jones and Bartlett's publications are available to corporations, professional associations, and other qualified organizations. For details and specific discount information, contact the special sales department at Jones and Bartlett via the above contact information or send an email to specialsales@jbpub.com.

The authors, editor, and publisher have made every effort to provide accurate information. However, they are not responsible for errors, omissions, or for any outcomes related to the use of the contents of this book and take no responsibility for the use of the products and procedures described. Treatments and side effects described in this book may not be applicable to all people; likewise, some people may require a dose or experience a side effect that is not described herein. Drugs and medical devices are discussed that may have limited availability controlled by the Food and Drug Administration (FDA) for use only in a research study or clinical trial. Research, clinical practice, and government regulations often change the accepted standard in this field. When consideration is being given to use of any drug in the clinical setting, the health care provider or reader is responsible for determining FDA status of the drug, reading the package insert, and reviewing prescribing information for the most up-to-date recommendations on dose, precautions, and contraindications, and determining the appropriate usage for the product. This is especially important in the case of drugs that are new or seldom used.

Dr. Kimball was an investigator and consultant for Galderma, Centocor, Amgen, Neostrata, and Abbott and an investigator for Stiefel within the year that this edition was revised.

Production Credits

Publisher: Christopher Davis
Editorial Assistant: Sara Cameron
Associate Production Editor: Sarah Bayle
Senior Marketing Manager: Barb Bartoszek
Manufacturing and Inventory Control Supervisor: Amy Bacus

Composition: Glyph International
Cover Design: Carolyn Downer
Cover Image: © William Casey/Shutterstock, Inc.; © Yori Arcurs, Shutterstock, Inc.
Printing and Binding: Malloy, Inc.
Cover Printing: Malloy, Inc.

Library of Congress Cataloging-in-Publication Data
Bergstrom, Kendra Gail.
    100 questions & answers about psoriasis / Kendra Gail Bergstrom, Alexa Boer Kimball.
        p. cm.
    Includes index.
    ISBN 978-0-7637-7735-7 (alk. paper)
    1. Psoriasis—Popular works. 2. Psoriasis—Miscellanea. I. Kimball, Alexa Boer. II. Title. III. Title: One hundred questions & answers about psoriasis. IV. Title: 100 questions and answers about psoriasis.
    RL321.B468 2010
    616.5'26—dc22
                                                                2009039588

6048
Printed in the United States of America
13 12 11 10 09   10 9 8 7 6 5 4 3 2 1

Contents

Part 5: Social Effects of Psoriasis 135

Psoriasis is one of the most common skin diseases in the United States. As many as 7.5 million people are affected by psoriasis and psoriatic arthritis in the United States alone. Approximately 1 out of every 50 adults will be affected by this disease at some point, and of these people, 1.5 million will suffer from moderate or severe psoriasis. Every year, approximately 200,000 new cases of psoriasis are diagnosed.

Psoriasis is not simply a disease of the skin. Although psoriasis does not cause life-threatening problems for the majority of patients, the effect on people's lives can be substantial and is often underestimated. This very visible disease can cause patients to feel self-conscious and ashamed about their appearance, which can lead to social isolation, psychological stress, or depression.

At present, psoriasis is a lifelong illness without a permanent cure. However, new therapies are being developed and innovative research continues in hopes of finding a cure. With an arsenal of topical steroids, topical and systemic immunosuppressants, novel biologics, and other treatments, patients now have a wider range of options than ever before. Even in the 5 years since the publication of our first edition, new therapies have been approved worldwide, and others have entered the pipeline. Many of these treatments are highly effective in controlling psoriasis and psoriatic arthritis and can alleviate the suffering often associated with this immune-mediated disease. Substantial progress has been made in understanding the complicated genetics and immunology that drive this disease, as well as identifying the other medical conditions that may be relevant for patients.

This book is designed to provide you with answers to many of the common questions we have found patients and their families ask about psoriasis. Although patients may feel overwhelmed at first by the experience of psoriasis, we hope that this book will offer information to alleviate some of that frustration. The most powerful weapon in the battle against any disease is understanding it, and we hope that this book will provide an initial step toward gaining knowledge.

Kendra Gail Bergstrom, MD
Alexa Boer Kimball, MD, MPH

Psoriasis is unpredictable. The person with psoriasis does not know when his disease will worsen or improve. He searches for patterns, but the stress of not being able to control his health can lead to anger and even hopelessness.

Psoriasis often carries a social stigma. The psoriasis patient may hide her skin to avoid stares and comments, wearing long sleeves and pants to summer picnics, and avoid photographs. Sometimes even family and friends make thoughtless comments.

Psoriasis is mysterious. Although it is the most common autoimmune disease, few people know about psoriasis and even fewer understand that it is a genetic, noncontagious disease affecting 7.5 million Americans.

Psoriasis and psoriatic arthritis are often undertreated. Research shows that more than 55% of people with psoriasis do not receive any treatment or their treatment does not do enough to relieve their symptoms. Many do not know that their psoriasis is also associated with increased risk of heart disease, hypertension, diabetes, and other serious conditions.

Psoriasis and psoriatic arthritis are serious and often debilitating diseases. The people who deal with them day in and day out need information, support, and action.

The National Psoriasis Foundation is a volunteer-driven nonprofit organization dedicated to improving the lives of people with psoriasis and psoriatic arthritis. In 2009, we created a new strategic plan outlining five major ways we will work to meet our mission.

Our highest priority is to find a cure for psoriasis. Hundreds of thousands of members, their families, and doctors are joining our community and working toward this goal.

Over the next 5 years we will increase the foundation's role as a catalyst in scientific discovery by investing in and encouraging research toward a cure. We will also continue to strengthen our presence as advocates by urging the passage of important legislation to increase research funding and improve access to care for people with psoriasis.

One of our most important strategic priorities is to increase the capacity of individuals and healthcare providers to effectively manage and treat psoriasis and psoriatic arthritis and improve overall health. This book, now in its second edition, has already helped countless patients, their families, and their doctors better understand this disease. We are grateful to Drs. Alexa Kimball and Kendra Bergstrom for providing an important resource for people with psoriasis.

Reading this book will help you understand your disease and take charge of your own health. Many more resources—including how to join us in our quest for a cure—are available from the National Psoriasis Foundation by calling (800) 723-9166 or visiting www.psoriasis.org.

Randy Beranek
President and CEO
National Psoriasis Foundation

PART ONE

The Basics

What is skin?

What is psoriasis?

How common is psoriasis?

More . . .

1. What is skin?

The **skin** is the largest organ in the body, covering 1.8 square meters of surface area. Over that area the skin senses temperature, pressure, and pain; conserves water; sweats to cool the body; and heals itself if injured or infected.

While many diseases such as acne or eczema primarily affect the skin, skin can also change because of diseases that affect other body systems. Before many of the present diagnostic tests were developed, physicians looked at the skin for information about the health of the entire body (**Figure 1**).

In addition to protecting, preserving water, and sensing for the body, the skin is presented to the world. Composed of the skin, hair, nails, and **mucous membranes**, the skin is a

Skin

The largest organ of the body, acting as a physically protective covering, site of the sense of touch, and a border of immune surveillance.

The skin is the largest organ in the body, covering 1.8 square meters of surface area.

Mucous membranes

The linings of the mouth, nose, vagina, and urethra (inside of the penis). These moist skin areas secrete mucus to keep the surfaces moist.

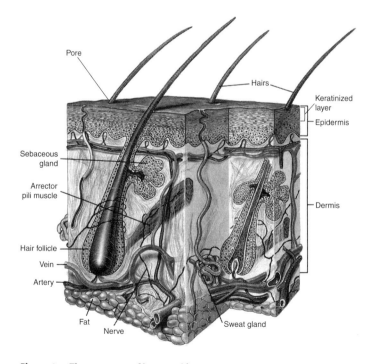

Figure 1   The structure of human skin.

tremendously important part of how we see ourselves and how others view us.

In a social environment, the skin is a large part of the interface between ourselves and the world. The skin gives signals about youth or age, and, along with the muscles of the face, expresses feelings. Because visual input is a significant part of communication, the skin's appearance can have a large impact on how people interact with each other.

The skin is organized into layers, and each level has a different function. The most superficial upper layer is called the **epidermis**, which contains **cells** that constitute the uppermost skin layer and cells that make pigment. This self-regenerating layer develops into the top layer of "skin cells" and the pigment that gives the skin its color. Pigment cells, or **melanocytes**, reside in the bottom layer of the epidermis, and when they are grouped together can appear as moles. The function of the epidermis is to be the front line of protection against water loss, physical stress, and **ultraviolet (UV) radiation**. The epidermis is especially thick on the palms and the soles of the feet and is often thickened in skin affected by psoriasis.

Deeper in the skin, the **dermis** contains the skin's blood vessels, nerves, hair follicles, sweat glands, and immune cells. The dermis provides nutrients to support the epidermis and nerves to sense physical contact and trauma. When a cut, scrape, burn, or crack breaks through the epidermis, the nerves, immune cells, and supportive parts of the dermis sense this break and cooperate to repair it. Blood vessels bring nutrients that feed the skin, and immune cells both fight infection and, in the case of psoriasis, cause skin inflammation.

The Basics

Epidermis

The outermost layer of skin. It is the non-vascular (without blood vessels) layer that covers and protects the dermis.

Cell

The basic structural and functional unit in the human body; the building blocks of each organ and tissue.

Melanocyte

The skin cell that produces melanin (the primary pigment that gives skin its color) and is found in the basal layer of the epidermis.

Ultraviolet (UV) radiation

Invisible rays that are part of the energy that comes from the sun. It is made up of two types of rays: UVA and UVB.

Dermis

The layer of skin just underneath the epidermis that contains the skin's nerve endings, blood vessels, hair follicles, sweat glands, and immune cells.

Systemic

Something that reaches or affects the entire body.

Immune system

The immune system is a collection of cells and proteins that works to protect the body from potentially harmful or infectious microorganisms such as bacteria, viruses, and fungi. The immune system plays a role in the control of cancer and other diseases, but can also cause autoimmune diseases, allergies, and rejection of transplanted organs.

White blood cell

A specialized type of cell present in the blood that works to fight against infection.

T cell

A type of white blood cell that attacks foreign and infected cells to protect the body.

B cell

A type of white blood cell in the blood and bone marrow that makes antibodies.

Although treating skin and the diseases that affect it can be particularly challenging, the treatment options are exceptionally varied. Unlike most organs, skin can be treated with locally acting topical medicines such as creams or ointments (see Question 34) that minimize **systemic** effects.

2. What is the immune system?

The **immune system** works to protect the body from infection. It monitors the body constantly and springs into action when it senses a foreign presence such as bacteria, a virus, or a fungus. In some situations, such as a cut or scrape, physical injury by itself is sufficient to set the immune system into action to protect against possible infection.

The immune system is comprised of a specialized group of cells and organs. Among the blood cells, the **white blood cells** are active in the immune system. Specialized white cells like **T cells, B cells**, and **neutrophils** (cells that make up pus) are important parts of the immune system. The immune system also has specialized locations in the body, including the lymph nodes and organs such as the spleen, thymus, tonsils, and appendix. The communication between these many cell types and organs is remarkable, and it occurs throughout the body through signals in the blood.

When the immune system is functioning properly, it guards against both external infections and internal damage. For example, the immune system watches for cells that could become cancer and tries to stop them. At times, however, the immune system is not watching closely enough and may miss a precancerous cell that later turns into cancer. At other times, though, the immune system may be watching too closely and decides that some part of the body—skin cells, or

4

keratinocytes, in the case of psoriasis—is not healthy or does not belong and may become activated.

3. What is psoriasis?

Psoriasis is a chronic, lifelong skin disease characterized by skin with white scale, redness, swelling, and itching or pain. It appears without a trigger or warning in the teens to 30s (for most people) and waxes and wanes in severity for life. Psoriasis is almost never fatal but can cause severe discomfort, disfigurement, and disability for sufferers. It can also be associated with a destructive form of arthritis.

Although the name psoriasis was not introduced for many years, the description of psoriasis and the beneficial effects of sunlight (which can ease psoriasis) were noted in the ancient Greek world. References to this skin disease are found in writings by the Greek physician Hippocrates, who lived from 460 to 377 BC. The English dermatologist Robert Willan, who lived from 1757 to 1812, was the first to recognize psoriasis as an independent disease. He described the scaly **plaques** of psoriasis as *leprosy graecorum*, an active, severe disease like *psora leprosa*, although there is no connection between psoriasis and leprosy.

In 1841, Ferdinand Hebra, a Viennese dermatologist working from Dr. Willan's notes, was the first to use the word "psoriasis" to describe the disease. Dr. Hebra first described the clinical picture of psoriasis that is used today. Hereditary associations in psoriasis had been established by this time.

The word psoriasis comes from the Greek psora, meaning itch or rash, and -iasis, a suffix that indicates a condition characterized or produced by an itch or

Neutrophil

The most common type of white blood cell in the bloodstream, it helps defend against bacterial infections. When these cells accumulate in large areas, pus is formed.

Keratinocyte

A skin cell of the epidermis that makes keratin, a protein that gives strength to skin, hair, and nails.

Plaque

In psoriasis, an area of skin affected by the disease.

The Basics

rash. Over the last century physicians have considered it a disease of skin differentiation (the way skin forms complete layers) and have developed therapies against scale and thickness. Recent research into the disease and therapy points toward an immune cause for the thickness, redness, and scaling of psoriasis. The immune system, when it is overactive in the skin, appears to cause changes in skin differentiation that lead to scaling and thickening. This new understanding of immune disruption in psoriasis has led to targeted therapies for the disease.

A formal description of psoriasis, developed by psoriasis experts at the American Academy of Dermatology, is "[a] chronic skin disease that is classically characterized by thickened, red areas of skin covered with silvery scale." In psoriatic skin (skin changed by psoriasis), plaques become red, thickened, or scaly and may be itchy or painful. The characteristics of a typical skin plaque depend on the type of psoriasis and body location affected. Psoriasis frequently affects the elbows, knees, scalp, and trunk. It may rarely appear on the hands and feet, mouth, skin folds, or genitals.

Psoriasis frequently affects the elbows, knees, scalp, and trunk.

When compared to other common skin diseases, such as eczema, psoriasis shows less swelling or oozing and a dry, white, shiny scale. Other skin diseases that can look similar to psoriasis include seborrheic dermatitis, pityriasis rosea, lichen planus, and skin forms of lupus.

A few characteristics of psoriasis have historically been used to diagnose the disease. These signs may be visible, especially in untreated psoriasis. **Auspitz's sign** is positive when the skin bleeds in pinpoint locations after peeling off a piece of scale from the skin. A positive Auspitz's sign is considered characteristic for

Auspitz's sign

A skin phenomenon, often seen in psoriasis, where pinpoint spots of blood appear when a scale is lifted off of the skin.

psoriasis because it does not occur after removing scale from other skin diseases. The **Woronoff ring** is seen in a ring of skin around the edges of a psoriasis plaque, when the surrounding unaffected skin becomes a paler, whiter color than the rest of the unaffected skin (see color plate A).

Some types of psoriasis appear different than the classic description. Other varieties include **inverse psoriasis** (affecting the skin folds), **guttate psoriasis** (in small spots all over the body; see color plate C), **palmar-plantar psoriasis** (on the hands and feet), **erythrodermic psoriasis** (where the entire body may turn red; see color plate D), and **pustular psoriasis** (with sterile, noninfected pustules). These varieties of psoriasis are caused by the same processes but appear as distinct forms of the disease. Because their locations and appearance are different, they may require different treatments for effective control.

4. What causes psoriasis?

The exact cause of psoriasis is still unknown. Two processes—rapid skin growth and inflammation—combine to cause the skin changes that lead to psoriasis. The initiating trigger for these processes—what makes the process begin in a particular person—remains obscure, and active research is ongoing to identify these events.

Under the microscope, skin affected by psoriasis is thicker than normal skin, with dramatic thickening of the epidermis (**hyperkeratinization**) and inflammation caused by a type of white blood cell called T cells. These T cells react against parts of the skin where the disease is active. The T cells and other immune system cells make cytokines, immune-system chemicals with names like TNFα (tumor necrosis factor alpha) and IL 23

Woronoff ring

A ring of pale-appearing skin that may be visible at the edge of a psoriasis plaque.

Inverse psoriasis

Psoriasis that affects skin folds, intertriginous areas, and/or genitals.

Guttate psoriasis

Psoriasis that appears as little drops scattered all over the skin (instead of fewer large plaques), sometimes associated with an infection.

Palmar-plantar psoriasis

Psoriasis on the hands and feet. This psoriasis may appear different from other types. (Also called palmoplantar psoriasis.)

Erythrodermic psoriasis

Full-body redness caused by psoriasis.

Pustular psoriasis

A type of psoriasis where sterile (uninfected) pustules appear on the skin.

Hyperkeratinization

Skin thickened in the outermost layer, caused by the overactivity of keratinocytes in psoriasis.

(interleukin 23), that aid in their communication and activation. Chronic inflammation in these areas causes skin cells to divide and turn over much more rapidly, up to four to five times as quickly as in normal skin. The rapid buildup of these skin cells, called keratinocytes, can lead to thick white scales on top of psoriatic skin. Over time, new, small blood vessels develop in the deeper layers of the skin. These blood vessels support the actively developing psoriatic plaques and may cause a persistent reddening of affected skin even after treatment. It is not yet clear why the T cells become activated in the skin in psoriasis and other immune diseases, but once the process starts, it seems to persist for life. How to inactivate or "turn off" these particular T cells permanently without impairing the immune system as a whole or causing serious **side effects** is a significant treatment challenge and is the focus of active immunology research.

Side effect

An undesired effect of a medication.

Gene

The segment of DNA on a chromosome that contains the information necessary to make a protein. A gene is the unit of biologic inheritance.

Studies of people and their relatives with psoriasis show that there is a genetic or familial predisposition to the disease, but not all people with certain **genes** or affected siblings will get the disease (discussed in Question 25). So far, most of the possible genes associated with psoriasis are part of the immune system. Different genes and groups of genes are more common in people with psoriasis, but most people with these genes do not develop psoriasis, and many people with psoriasis do not have these genes. Some researchers have found that you need to have a group of relatively common genes to be susceptible. One gene that seems consistently important, however, is called HLA-C. For these reasons, genetic testing is only used for research at this point and cannot offer useful information about psoriasis diagnosis, treatment, or prognosis.

Active research into the cause of psoriasis has shown that certain immune system genes are associated with this and other immune processes. The next step, using this information to develop new therapies, is underway.

5. How common is psoriasis?

Statistics vary, but current estimates indicate that 2% to 3% of the U.S. population, or around 5 to 7 million adults, have some psoriasis on their skin. Approximately 200,000 people are newly diagnosed with psoriasis each year. The prevalence rate varies in different ethnic groups and is higher in Caucasians than in blacks, Hispanics, Asians, and Native Americans. The reasons for different prevalence rates are not known but are believed to be due to the association with certain genetic backgrounds (discussed in Question 25).

Because psoriasis appears for the first time in the majority of people while in their 20s, it is found less often in children, and new diagnoses are even rarer in older people. Because psoriasis is less common in children and older people, a psoriasis diagnosis in these individuals may not be immediately clear.

Among people who have psoriasis, **psoriasis vulgaris** (vulgaris meaning common), or **plaque psoriasis**, is the most common form, found in over 85% of people with psoriasis (see color plate G). The other types of psoriasis comprise around 15% of cases, though people may have more than one type at the same time. One type of psoriasis, guttate psoriasis, is more commonly found in children after a throat, skin, or other infection and sometimes resolves after the infection is treated. Because these rarer types of psoriasis look different than the common type, they may be undiagnosed or misdiagnosed in some individuals for a period of time.

The Basics

Psoriasis vulgaris

The most common form of psoriasis, it usually appears as scaly, red plaques on the elbows, knees, and scalp.

Plaque psoriasis

The most common form of psoriasis, also called psoriasis vulgaris.

The incidence of psoriasis worldwide varies somewhat but is generally in the 2% to 5% range. The highest incidence is estimated at 10% among people from northern Europe and is the lowest in parts of South America and Samoa where no psoriasis has been reported. Women and men are equally affected by psoriasis.

Women and men are equally affected by psoriasis.

For people with psoriasis, approximately 5% to 30% may develop **psoriatic arthritis**, and this is more likely to occur in people with more severe disease. For most people, arthritis appears 5 to 10 years after skin psoriasis, though in a small group of people it may be the first sign of psoriasis.

Psoriatic arthritis

A term for the several types of arthritis that can develop in people with psoriasis. It is distinct from other common types of arthritis and may need to be treated differently.

John's comment:

Most people tend to hide their psoriasis, and accordingly, it seems like I am the only person in the world with psoriasis. It is great to know that I am not alone. There are probably more people in the United States with psoriasis than inhabitants of Los Angeles. I just wish we were all more open about it, so it might become more accepted and better understood by society at large.

6. Who gets psoriasis?

Any person can develop psoriasis. This common skin condition does not spare any gender, ethnicity, or those with other skin diseases. For most people, psoriasis is diagnosed in their teens or 20s. Men and women are equally affected. Some children may be diagnosed with psoriasis, but the disease may look different from adult psoriasis.

Some people are at increased risk for psoriasis. Specifically, a person's risk increases if a first-degree relative (parent, grandparent, or sibling) has psoriasis. Other risk factors for psoriasis include psoriasis in other family members (aunts, uncles, and cousins), psoriatic arthritis in family members, or a family history of autoimmune diseases. When people with psoriasis are surveyed about having family members with the disease, 40% to 65% of individuals know of an affected family member.

Many studies have investigated how a person's genetic background affects psoriasis. The genes that seem to be common in psoriasis sufferers—and less common in people without psoriasis—are those in the immune system. Although this information may be therapeutically useful in the future, at the present time no test is commercially available to determine the genotype or genetic fingerprint of psoriasis sufferers, and no changes in prognosis or therapy would be needed based on the results.

In studies of siblings, twins, and first-degree relatives (siblings, parents, and children), relative risks have been estimated. When one twin has psoriasis, the chance of the second twin being diagnosed was 58% in one study, based on 141 sets of twins. If a sibling has psoriasis, the chance of another sibling developing the disease is lower, around 6%. When one parent has psoriasis, the chance of a child acquiring the disease is below 20%, but if both parents have psoriasis the chance increases to 65%. The severity of disease varies within families, and not every related person with psoriasis has the same amount or location of the disease.

7. Why does a person get psoriasis?

Aside from an association with some immune system genes, the reason an individual gets psoriasis is not known. Studies to date have investigated the role of bacteria, viruses, and environmental triggers without conclusive answers.

Although the questions "Why me?" or "Why anyone?" can't be answered at this time, no action, or lack of action currently identified, can control whether psoriasis appears.

Many influences such as stress, medications, and skin trauma are known to exacerbate psoriasis, yet none of these influences by themselves or in combination are known to cause psoriasis. The initial triggers for psoriasis are not known and are not preventable at this time. Mitigating stress is a challenging project, but one that is known to help psoriasis and many other autoimmune diseases.

Many scientists have tried to pinpoint the immunologic trigger that begins the psoriasis process. Some researchers believe that a bacterial protein or fungus may be a trigger, and others believe that skin trauma may instigate and worsen psoriasis. No one entity appears to be the culprit in the majority of cases, and at this point, none of these theories have been proven or disproved.

One exception is guttate psoriasis, especially in children. This less common type of psoriasis may be triggered by a skin, throat, or ear infection, usually with the Streptococcus bacteria, commonly known as "strep." Guttate psoriasis sometimes resolves with treatment of the initial infection. Guttate psoriasis triggered by an infection is usually distinctive because of the specific pattern of small (0.25 to 0.5 inch [0.5 to 1.0 cm] in diameter) spots all over the body, usually appearing in childhood or young adulthood. Some people who have had guttate psoriasis will go on to develop the more common form of plaque psoriasis.

8. How is psoriasis diagnosed?

Psoriasis is often diagnosed by a **dermatologist** or primary care physician by its characteristic appearance and locations on the body. If a person has the skin changes typical of psoriasis, a diagnosis can be made clinically by examination alone. Based on the skin's appearance due to psoriasis, a physician will usually be able to diagnose psoriasis and begin treating the skin immediately.

If psoriasis looks different than most cases, appears in an unusual location, or appears in a child, further tests may be needed. The definitive test when a **clinical diagnosis** of skin disease is unclear is a **skin biopsy**. A biopsy refers to a small sample of skin taken for analysis under a microscope. For a biopsy, a small sample of skin (about a 0.25-inch [4-mm] core, the size of a pencil eraser) is removed for examination under the microscope by a **dermatopathologist**. A dermatopathologist is a physician who specializes in analyzing skin samples under the microscope for diagnostic clues. The findings of the dermatopathologist are summarized in a **pathology report**. Usually, only one test is required, but it may be repeated if the results aren't clear or if the disease changes over time. A person can request a copy of this report for his or her records, and most physicians will find it useful to review it when planning treatment (discussed in Question 18).

No blood test exists to diagnose psoriasis, and psoriasis does not cause abnormal blood tests for most people. The most common reason to draw blood when treating people for psoriasis is to make sure it is safe to begin a

The Basics

Dermatologist

A physician specializing in the diagnosis and treatment of skin disease.

Clinical diagnosis

Diagnosis based on clinical information, such as appearance and history, as opposed to being based on laboratory tests.

Skin biopsy

The surgical removal of a piece of skin (often the size of a pencil eraser) for examination under a microscope. A biopsy is often done to diagnose a skin disease.

Dermatopathologist

A physician specializing in diagnosing skin disease by its appearance under the microscope.

Pathology report

The formal report of a physician after looking at a skin sample under the microscope. This report is part of a patient's medical record.

new medication or to watch for a medicine's possible side effects. One exception is severe psoriasis covering much of the body, where changes in the skin's barrier function could cause dehydration or salt imbalances.

If a person has joint pain or swelling anywhere in the body, evaluation for psoriatic arthritis is essential. This diagnosis may be made by a dermatologist, **rheumatologist**, **orthopedist**, or other joint specialist. The evaluation for psoriatic arthritis may include X-rays, joint tests, and blood panels to look for other causes of arthritis. It is important to consider a possible diagnosis of psoriatic arthritis in any person with psoriasis. To minimize the risk of permanent joint damage, prompt follow-up with appropriate tests for accurate diagnosis and treatment is important.

9. Is psoriasis contagious?

One of the most common misconceptions about psoriasis is that it is a contagious disease. Much of the uncertainty and fear people experience when seeing psoriasis for the first time comes from a fear of "catching it." Psoriasis is not contagious and has no infectious component. No amount of skin-to-skin contact, caring for another person's affected skin, or sharing of personal items such as towels or cups causes the transmission of psoriasis. Because there is no infectious cause, and the disease is caused by the white blood cells inside a person's own body, no transmission is possible.

Some psoriasis sufferers find it helpful to briefly explain what psoriasis is and why it is not contagious. People who don't understand the disease may confuse any rash with contagious infections like skin fungus (such as ringworm, athlete's foot, or jock itch),

Rheumatologist

A physician who specializes in diseases of the immune system and the joints.

Orthopedist

A surgeon concerned with the diagnosis, care, and treatment of musculoskeletal disorders. (Also known as orthopedic surgeon.)

One of the most common misconceptions about psoriasis is that it is a contagious disease.

14

impetigo (staph or strep infections of the skin), eczema, rashes due to viral infections, infestations such as mites or scabies, or even an imagined skin disease.

If one person in a family has psoriasis and others are diagnosed with the disease later, the cause is thought to stem from a shared genetic predisposition and has no relation to physical contact. Families can be reassured that physical contact with their loved ones is welcome and helpful for most psoriasis sufferers.

The question of possible infection or contagiousness is a common one, and can be a source of much anxiety for sufferers and nonsufferers alike. Correct information about psoriasis, for family and friends as well as the community, can alleviate some of the misdirected fear associated with the disease.

Psoriasis sufferers can prepare themselves with knowledge and techniques to explain the noninfectious cause of the disease. Organizations such as the **National Psoriasis Foundation** have suggestions for talking about psoriasis for people of all ages. Clearing up this common misconception is often the most effective first step in talking about psoriasis.

National Psoriasis Foundation
The largest not-for-profit national organization dedicated to helping people with psoriasis.

Although psoriasis is not contagious, it can spread and affect different parts of the skin. Psoriasis may begin anywhere on the body, but the most common places it appears and spreads are predictable. While every person is different, most people notice a similar pattern. The most common type of psoriasis, psoriasis vulgaris, has a characteristic appearance pattern on the elbows, knees, scalp, and trunk (**Figure 2**; see also color plates A, B, and F).

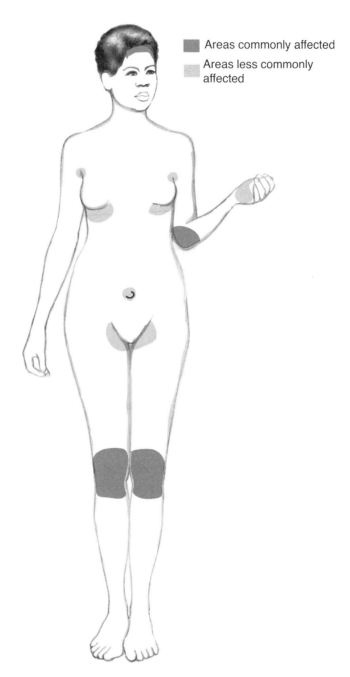

Areas commonly affected

Areas less commonly affected

Figure 2   Psoriasis vulgaris is most commonly located on the elbows, knees, scalp, and trunk.

When a person has psoriasis in one location, a physician will usually check these common locations to see if psoriasis is present elsewhere. It can also appear any place the skin has experienced trauma, such as an old scar or new skin injury (discussed in Question 30). For most people, psoriasis appears in a symmetric pattern, though some may have only one or two areas of psoriasis on the skin.

Although the majority of people have a typical pattern of plaque psoriasis, some people will have different types of psoriasis. Places where psoriasis may appear in a less common pattern include the skin folds under the armpits (see color plate H) and in the groin. This is called **intertriginous psoriasis** or inverse psoriasis. Other types include palmar-plantar psoriasis, guttate psoriasis, pustular psoriasis, and erythrodermic psoriasis. Typically, only one type of psoriasis is present in an individual, though overlapping types may occur.

Intertriginous psoriasis

Psoriasis that affects intertriginous areas such as the armpits or the groin. This type of psoriasis can appear different than other types of psoriasis and may be treated differently.

In severe cases, psoriasis can spread to cover the entire body. When psoriasis causes redness covering over 90% of the body, it is called erythrodermic psoriasis, a serious and possibly life-threatening condition. The involvement of the entire skin area impairs the body's ability to fight off infection and keep moisture inside the skin barrier, and can increase the risk of infection. Depending on the severity of the psoriasis and a person's overall health, this condition may warrant a hospital stay for monitoring and treatment.

John's comment:

Thankfully it is not contagious. This fact is the foundation of being able to participate in society. It would be great if everyone in the United States knew this without having to mention it.

10. Can psoriasis be cured?

At this time, no cure exists for psoriasis. Like many immune-mediated diseases, it is treated with therapies that decrease immune activity. Unfortunately, no current treatment decreases the activity of the immune cells permanently. Current therapies suppress the signs and symptoms of psoriasis but are unable to treat the ultimate cause—activation of the immune system in the skin.

In most people, psoriasis waxes and wanes with time. Many people experience periods of time where it is gone completely. For almost all sufferers, however, the disease does return. Because the immune system is primed to react in the skin, it continues to do so over time.

Many different "miracle" therapies and "cures" have been advertised for psoriasis. However, because psoriasis has multiple causes, and the immune system cannot be easily retrained, most people will need to be treated on an ongoing basis. Therefore, while many therapies are effective to calm the symptoms of psoriasis, claims of a cure must be evaluated with great care.

A realistic goal for most people is to find a personal balance between control of their psoriasis and the amount of time, effort, and expense they want to invest in treatments. Because all medications carry some risk, the balance between effectiveness and side effects must also be evaluated carefully.

There is hope that, in the future, a cure will be found. Active research is being done by immunologists and skin biologists, and applied research is being undertaken by academic medical centers and pharmaceutical companies. Psoriasis remains a priority of researchers, and new developments and discoveries continue to unfold.

11. What else besides skin is affected by psoriasis?

For most people, the skin is the only manifestation of their psoriasis. However, it is useful to be aware of less common manifestations of psoriasis that occur elsewhere in the body. Aside from the more common nail psoriasis and psoriatic arthritis, there are other places that psoriasis may rarely appear.

Mucous Membranes

Psoriasis sometimes affects the mucous membranes of the lips, inside of the mouth, and the tongue. In rare cases, people may have psoriasis on or in the mouth. When psoriasis is on the tongue, it may have jagged borders separating areas of lighter and darker color, much like a map. This characteristic appearance has led to the term "**geographic tongue**," which can happen in people with or without psoriasis.

Joints

The joints, especially those in the hands, may be affected by psoriasis in a specialized form of arthritis called psoriatic arthritis (discussed in Question 20).

Eyes

In rare cases, psoriasis can cause a red, painful ring around the pupil of the eye in a condition called **iritis** or anterior uveitis. It has been reported rarely as a presenting symptom of psoriasis and can be diagnosed by an ophthalmologist.

Geographic tongue

Geographic tongue describes a map-like appearance of the tongue. This results from irregular, denuded patches on its surface. It is not painful and can be found in healthy people.

Iritis

Inflammation of the eye, sometimes as the result of an autoimmune disease. Also called anterior uveitis.

Other conditions associated with psoriasis are discussed in Question 17.

12. What causes psoriasis to get worse?

The course of psoriasis is different in each person. Some people find that their psoriasis is cyclical (following seasons of the year or other events), and others find the disease unremitting and constant over time. In some individuals, the skin may worsen at certain times. Although every person's skin reacts differently, exacerbating factors, including changes in medications and stress, are common among many patients.

Harold's comment:

My psoriasis seems to get worse when I'm under stress, the weather is dry, and if I fail to keep moisturizer or medicines applied to it.

Stress

Both emotional and physical stress can cause psoriasis to flare or worsen.

Both emotional and physical stress can cause psoriasis to flare or worsen. A psoriasis flare could occur weeks or months after a stressful event. Stressful events can range from major life changes, such as the death of a family member or a job change, to a new diet or the flu. Some people find it helpful to practice stress-reduction techniques, whether it's yoga or meditation or spending time with family or a pet. Although illness and other stressful events are at times unavoidable, a careful eye on psoriatic skin can pick up exacerbations early and treat them aggressively (discussed in Question 93).

Medications

Any medication (or changing medications) can affect the skin. In particular, classes of medications known to cause psoriasis flares include the following (discussed at length in Question 75):

Medications for high blood pressure:

- Thiazide diuretics (e.g., hydrochlorothiazide)
- Beta-blockers (e.g., metoprolol, propranolol, atenolol, and labetolol)
- Calcium channel blockers (e.g., amlodipine, verapamil, and diltiazem)
- ACE inhibitors (e.g., captopril and enalapril)

Other medications:

- Oral steroids when suddenly stopped (**prednisone** and dexamethasone)
- **Nonsteroidal anti-inflammatories** (Ibuprofen and naproxen)
- Immune system stimulators (GM-CSF)
- Antimalarials (chloroquine)
- Lithium

These medications do not cause flares in all people. However, if psoriasis worsens after starting one of these medicines, consider discussing with a doctor whether an alternative medication could be used in its place.

For any medication, if psoriasis worsens after beginning or increasing a dose, consider following the same steps. However, for new medications, such as antibiotics prescribed to treat an infection, it is important to consider whether the underlying problem might be the trigger for a psoriasis flare.

Fall and Winter

Because sunlight helps calm psoriasis, the decrease in sunlight hours during the fall and winter can worsen

Prednisone

A type of cortisone (a so-called "stress hormone" naturally made by the body) that can be taken by mouth.

Nonsteroidal anti-inflammatories (NSAIDs)

Aspirin, ibuprofen (the active ingredient in Motrin or Advil), indomethacin, and some other painkillers have both anti-inflammatory and anti-pain properties. These medications are distinct from steroid-based anti-inflammatories such as prednisone and dexamethasone, and distinct from acetaminophen (Tylenol).

PUVA

The use of psoralen medication, by mouth or on the skin, combined with UVA light to treat psoriasis.

UVB

A particular wavelength of light that is used in combination with a medication called psoralen to treat psoriasis.

Koebner phenomenon

This phenomenon, seen in psoriasis and other skin diseases, occurs when skin trauma initiates new lesions in previously healthy skin. Also referred to as Koebnerization.

Phototherapy

The use of light, whether from the sun or special light sources, to treat skin disease.

psoriasis. For people who respond well to sunlight, treatment with light therapy such as **PUVA** or **UVB** over the winter can supplement sunlight to the level available during the summer months (discussed in Question 56).

Skin Trauma

Psoriasis has a propensity to affect previously injured skin, an event named the **Koebner phenomenon** or Koebnerization (discussed in Question 30). The result is that injured skin anywhere on the body, whether damaged from surgical scars, tattoos, or even cosmetic procedures such as laser treatment or dermabrasion, may develop psoriasis even in unexpected areas. Although sun is beneficial to psoriasis, sunburn can worsen psoriasis through this phenomenon, whether the burn stems from natural sunlight, tanning beds, or **phototherapy** (discussed in Question 59).

Over time, many people notice cycles in the severity of their psoriasis and are able to predict which events, medications, or foods worsen their disease. Something that causes a severe flare in one person may not affect another. Because the triggers for worsening psoriasis are widely variable in different people, the best predictor for an individual's skin disease may be personal experience.

When trying to determine which factors seem to make skin better or worse, a diary can help to associate symptoms and events. A diary can include any important factors, typically psoriasis activity, treatment and medications, and daily routines such as diet, exercise, and daily activities. This recordkeeping can help to identify flare triggers and can track how changes in daily routine (such as a change in diet, for example) affect the skin.

13. How bad can psoriasis get?

John's comment:

Bad enough that I had severe pain when I walked due to psoriasis on the bottom of my feet, bad enough that I had severe pain when water ran against my fingers that were raw from psoriasis, bad enough that my nails were so brittle and fragile they were easily susceptible to breaking and exposing the nail bed, not to mention the disfiguring effect that I've had on my face, ears, nails, arms, legs, hands, feet, and other locations, sometimes with pain, sometimes with bleeding. There is also the driving itch—more compelling than a nicotine addiction.

Psoriasis, in its most severe form, may turn the skin red all over the body (erythrodermic psoriasis) or cause pustules to appear (pustular psoriasis). Erythrodermic psoriasis is named because the redness (erythro-) covers the entire body (dermic). This condition is rare but can be very serious. When psoriasis covers the entire body, in addition to discomfort and irritation, the skin's protective barrier breaks down. The skin may lose its ability to keep the body from losing water or protect from infection, and sufferers can become dehydrated or acquire an infection that could spread all over the body. When psoriasis is this severe, an individual may need to be admitted to a hospital for fluid infusion, psoriasis treatment, and careful observation to see if the disease improves. Pustular psoriasis can be equally severe.

These types of psoriasis are very rare, with erythrodermic psoriasis appearing in only 1% to 4% of people with psoriasis and serious pustular psoriasis in only 0.5% to 2%.

Historically, these severe exacerbations were more common before the current range of treatment options became available. The many immunosuppressive medications have allowed physicians to control psoriasis better and more rapidly, helping to prevent this kind of severe disease. Although it is difficult to predict who will experience a serious flare, those with more severe disease are also at a higher risk of **complications**. If a person has been using oral steroids such as prednisone for any reason and stops quickly, a severe form of psoriasis may develop when **steroids** are stopped. For this reason, those with psoriasis should take oral steroids with caution and should watch the skin carefully when the dose is lowered, tapered, or discontinued.

Most people with psoriasis will never have to worry about rare types of psoriasis. However, it is important to be aware of skin changes that may need immediate attention and treatment.

Sue's comment:

Showering was a really difficult experience. My skin burned—like pouring vinegar on an open wound—when the water hit my skin. My scalp and under my breasts were the worst. I would cry. Drying after the shower was just as painful. Sleeping was awful. I would itch all throughout the night. When I would drift off to sleep I would be awakened by pain because I'd moved my leg or my arm. I ached constantly.

14. What are common reactions to being diagnosed with psoriasis?

When first diagnosed with psoriasis, different people have different reactions. Anxiety, anger, and fear are not

Complication

A problem that occurs after using a medication or therapy. Also known as a side effect.

Steroid

A large class of pharmaceutical agents that chemically resemble cholesterol. Two well-known types are glucocorticoid steroids, used to reduce inflammation, and anabolic steroids, which are often used (illegally) in athletics.

uncommon. Some people may find relief at being able to name and understand their particular skin disease. Most people want to learn more about the disease and its management.

Psoriasis is at present a lifelong disease, and the news that this skin disease cannot currently be cured can be unexpected and upsetting. Understanding and accepting the prospect of managing this chronic skin disease is a lifelong process.

Because the disease is often diagnosed in adolescence or young adulthood, a feeling of alienation and loneliness is common. Some find relief at being able to name and understand their skin disease, but many people feel angry and frustrated with the new diagnosis or slow treatment results. Because skin is so visible, people may feel self-conscious at looking different.

Some people may want to hide their disease. Others may want to read as much as possible about it and therapy options. Many find it helpful to get in touch with other psoriasis sufferers through resources such as the National Psoriasis Foundation (discussed in Questions 86 and the Appendix). For children with psoriasis and other skin diseases, summer camps are available around the country that allow them to spend a week with others without feeling different because of their skin.

Common worries among psoriasis sufferers include social interaction with friends and loved ones, the possibility of passing on psoriasis to children, the cost and time involved in treatment, and the ability to continue all of the activities in daily life. The availability and cost of medical care may also be a concern. Others may worry about arthritis or other complications in the future.

Over-the-counter (OTC)

Products (medications, creams, vitamins, supplements, etc.) available at the drugstore. These medications can be effective but are not usually covered by medical insurance.

For a person newly diagnosed with psoriasis, talking with other people who have psoriasis can be an excellent starting point. Education, information, and connecting with others are an ideal way to begin.

15. Why do people keep talking about the "heartbreak of psoriasis"?

"Do you suffer from the heartbreak of psoriasis?" An advertising campaign in the early 1970s used that question in TV commercials to advertise a commonly used **over-the-counter (OTC)** topical steroid. For those who know little about the disease, this may be their only point of reference. Since then, treatments have improved to mitigate this "heartbreak," but the phrase has lived on to spawn numerous articles, commentaries, and even the name for a 1970s rock band. The reference sometimes reemerges in newer marketing campaigns for psoriasis treatments.

Heartbreak, while a dramatic term, does illustrate the inherent challenge of psoriasis. Psoriasis is almost never fatal but can be very upsetting to a person's life and self-image. The "heartbreak" label is, of course, subjective. A disease such as psoriasis, which may be devastating at one point in time, can be treated and is compatible with a long and healthy life. Moreover, improvements in treatment over the past decades and increased understanding of the disease have helped many people since this slogan was first coined.

PART TWO

Diagnosis

How does someone know whether he or
she has psoriasis?

If I have psoriasis, am I at risk for other
diseases as well?

What are the different types of psoriatic arthritis?

More . . .

16. How does someone know whether he or she has psoriasis?

Psoriasis is usually diagnosed by a general practitioner or dermatologist. It is most often a clinical diagnosis, meaning that the physical examination findings alone make the diagnosis clear. In different people, psoriasis tends to show similar skin changes, such as redness, thick skin, scaling, itching, and pain, and appear in the same areas (elbows, knees, and scalp, among others). When the clinical diagnosis is clear, a person will often need no laboratory tests. There are no blood tests needed to diagnose or treat psoriasis, however, blood tests may be used to monitor medications or to check for joint disease activity.

At times, the diagnosis of psoriasis may be unclear. This uncertainty may arise because skin changes appear in unexpected areas, look unusual, or are infected. When the diagnosis is not obvious, a physician will often need to sample the skin with a skin biopsy, a procedure that is usually performed by a dermatologist.

After diagnosis, a patient may be referred to a dermatologist for continuing care and treatment adjustments. A dermatologist's input is especially important if psoriasis is severe, hard to treat, changes unexpectedly, or causes a great deal of distress to the patient.

17. If I have psoriasis, am I at risk for other diseases as well?

People with psoriasis have a substantially increased risk for a particular type of joint disease called psoriatic arthritis. This type of arthritis, specific to psoriasis sufferers, causes pain, swelling, and joint destruction in a distinct pattern. Many people also have osteoarthritis (degenerative arthritis, the most common type, comes from the normal wear and tear on the joints over time) or, more rarely, rheumatoid arthritis. Psoriatic arthritis can have a different set of symptoms and is sometimes treated differently. Approximately 5% to 30% of people with psoriasis will get psoriatic arthritis; the risk of arthritis increases with more extensive skin disease.

Research has shown that people with psoriasis are at higher risk for high blood pressure, heart failure, diabetes, depression, alcoholism, and heart attack. One theory is that heart disease may be influenced by inflammation and the amount of inflammation in skin with psoriasis can be substantial. Psoriatics are also at risk for obesity, which can contribute to the risk of heart disease. **Crohn's disease**, a disease of the intestine, is also associated with psoriasis. Skin cancer can also be a side effect, especially for patients who have used light therapy or have taken immunosuppressing medications such as cyclosporine. This risk appears of be highest for people who have used PUVA treatment for psoriasis. One recent publication from Great Britain suggested that people with moderate or severe psoriasis have a small but increased lifetime risk of cancers of the blood, such as leukemia and lymphoma. This risk appears to be independent of the type and duration of treatments used for the disease. The lymphoma risk was low but increased for all psoriasis sufferers in this specific group of people with moderate or severe psoriasis, regardless of which treatments they had received.

One other risk of psoriasis is related to the medications used for treatment. All medications have potential side effects, or unwanted effects that can occur in the course of treating psoriasis. In particular, oral, **subcutaneous**

Crohn's disease
A chronic illness that causes irritation in the digestive tract. It occurs most commonly in the ileum (lower small intestine) or in the colon (large intestine).

Research has shown that people with psoriasis are at higher risk for high blood pressure, heart failure, diabetes, depression, alcoholism, and heart attack.

Subcutaneous
The tissue just below the surface of the skin. Some medicines are injected into this area.

Intravenous

Medication or fluid given by injection or infusion into a vein.

Biologic therapy

Medical therapy that is derived from a biologic source rather than being synthesized from a chemical source.

Immunosuppression

Suppression of the natural immune response because immune system defenses have been suppressed, damaged, or weakened.

PPD test

A skin test for previous exposure to tuberculosis. Certain tuberculosis proteins are injected under the skin, and after a few days the skin is checked to see if the body mounts a response (shown as a raised, red wheal).

Shave biopsy

A biopsy performed with a razor by cutting off a superficial piece of the skin.

(injected beneath the skin), and **intravenous** (injected into veins) medications may affect other parts of the body besides the skin. The presence and severity of these effects are usually related to dose level or total amount taken, but can appear unexpectedly at any time.

Most systemic treatments for psoriasis, such as prednisone, cyclosporine, methotrexate, and **biologic therapies**, work by suppressing the immune system. This medicine-induced **immunosuppression** puts people at increased risk for new infections or reactivation of old infections. One major concern of suppressing the immune system is reactivation of latent tuberculosis. If a person has been exposed to tuberculosis in the past, whether they know it or not, they may have successfully contained all infection in one location, usually the lung. Immunosuppressive medicines can reduce control of infection and allow tuberculosis to reactivate in the lung or other parts of the body. To minimize this risk, a physician will often do a tuberculosis test called a **PPD test** and/or a chest x-ray prior to beginning these therapies.

18. If I have a biopsy, how do I interpret the results?

A skin biopsy is a small sample of skin that is examined under the microscope to help diagnose a disease. Reasons to take a biopsy include evaluating a puzzling skin problem, removing or sampling a skin change suspicious for cancer, or removing a suspicious mole. Two types of skin biopsies are commonly done—a **shave biopsy** and a **punch biopsy**. A shave biopsy is performed with a sterile razor-like tool that is used to cuts off a superficial piece of the skin. The skin is then usually covered and left to heal itself. A punch biopsy uses a small, specially designed punching tool shaped like a miniature "cookie cutter." This punch is usually deeper than a shave and lets the examining physician see farther down into the skin. This is especially helpful if the skin is thick or the changes are deep in the skin. Because a punch biopsy is deeper than a shave biopsy, the punch is usually closed with small stitches or **sutures**. These sutures may dissolve in the skin or they may need to be removed. Different sutures are used and are left in for varying lengths of time depending on the thickness of the skin and the movement in the area. It is important to have a suture removed at the correct time to prevent scarring or reopening of a wound. For all biopsies, the skin is prepared by careful cleaning to reduce the risk of infection and is numbed to minimize discomfort.

After a biopsy is taken, the skin sample is preserved, cut into thin slices, and stained with special dyes to see differences in the tissue under the microscope. The biopsy results may return in 1 to 6 weeks, depending on the laboratory involved. If a result is still unclear or confusing, it may be sent to additional physicians for analysis. The results of a biopsy are usually formally reported in your medical chart at the doctor's office. When the results are available, you may consider keeping a copy with your personal medical record in case you see a different physician in the future.

19. What information should I bring to my dermatologist appointment?

Harold's comment:

Bring a family history, general health history and info on current conditions, a good sense of humor, and a clean pair of underwear!

Punch biopsy

A biopsy that uses a small, specially designed punching tool shaped like a miniature "cookie cutter." This punch is usually deeper than a shave and lets the examining physician see farther down into the skin.

Suture

A medical term for a stitch. Some sutures may need to be removed, while others can dissolve on their own.

Diagnosis

At a first visit with a dermatologist, the doctor will want to review a patient's skin history, medical and surgical history, and family history, and conduct a careful skin examination in one short visit; there's a lot of ground to cover.

In particular, you may be asked about the following:

Skin disease:

- A narrative of the development of your skin disease
- How it has changed over time
- What you have done to treat it up to this point

Medical history, including:

- Allergies to medications
- Chronic diseases, including liver disease and kidney disease
- History of skin disease, including symptoms of dandruff, itching, or skin cancer
- History of joint problems
- Medication history, especially for chronic medications

Tip: For any doctor's appointment, it's always a good idea to bring in a list of the medications or the medications themselves to make sure everything is up to date. Bringing the skin care products you use can also be helpful since moisturizers are an important part of maintenance.

Family history, including:

- Psoriasis
- Arthritis
- Skin cancer

Recent changes in health, including:

- Recent infections of the skin or anywhere else on the body
- Stressful life events
- New medications

Your thoughts on the disease and its treatment, including:

- Which aspect of the disease (appearance or itch, for example) is most worrisome to you?
- How aggressive do you want to be with treatment? How much time and money do you want to dedicate to the process?
- All therapies have side effects; what types of side effects are you most concerned about?

It's a good idea to collect this information ahead of time and consider your treatment preference before your visit. This information, together with the appearance of your skin, helps to guide a treatment plan. The approaches to treating psoriasis are many, and their effectiveness varies from person to person. Because of the chronic nature of psoriasis and the sometimes constant need for treatment, understanding an individual's background and thoughts about the skin is essential to make and refine a therapeutic plan.

The approaches to treating psoriasis are many, and their effectiveness varies from person to person.

20. My doctor told me I have psoriatic arthritis. How is this different from other types of arthritis?

Psoriatic arthritis is caused by the same inflammatory process that causes psoriasis of the skin. Because of joint pain, joint swelling, and a warm feeling to the touch, it may resemble other types of arthritis, particularly rheumatoid arthritis. Between 5% and 30% of people with psoriasis will get psoriatic arthritis, usually following skin disease by 5 to 10 years. However, it can be the first symptom of psoriasis, in which case it needs to be carefully differentiated from other types of arthritis.

It is important to distinguish psoriatic arthritis from rheumatoid arthritis, osteoarthritis, and other forms of arthritis because the course of the disease and its treatment may differ. A physician may recognize the symptoms of psoriatic arthritis as a clinical diagnosis, but the consultation of a rheumatologist, orthopedist, or other joint specialist is sometimes needed. The most common type of arthritis in most people, including those with psoriasis, is osteoarthritis. Unlike psoriatic arthritis, which is often the worst in the morning, osteoarthritis is usually worse at the end of the day after hours of using the joints.

Depending on the severity of your disease, you may have x-rays taken of the affected joints. These x-rays are helpful to determine how the joints look at diagnosis and to look for changes over time.

There are fairly recently developed criteria now published that are being used to diagnose psoriatic arthritis. One of these systems is the CASPAR criteria. The CASPAR criteria are met when a patient has established inflammatory joint disease and scores at least three points from the following list:

- Current psoriasis (scores two points)
- A history of psoriasis (unless current psoriasis was present), a family history of psoriasis (unless current psoriasis was present or there was a history of

psoriasis), dactylitis (swelling of fingers or toes), juxtaarticular new bone formation, rheumatoid factor negativity, and nail dystrophy (each scores one point).

Which joints are affected?

Joint disease is not necessarily determined by skin disease. That is, a joint directly beneath an affected skin area will not necessarily be involved. Joints that are often involved include the joints of the hands and fingers, the lower back (especially the **sacroiliac joint**, where the back meets the hips), and less commonly the knees, hips, or shoulders.

Who gets joint disease?

Studies suggest that people with nail changes in psoriasis, such as **oil spots** or **onycholysis**, are more likely to have joint disease. In different studies in the United States and worldwide, 35% of patients with psoriatic nails had this type of arthritis. People with more severe skin disease are also at increased risk, although the severity of the two conditions may vary considerably in an individual.

Therapy for psoriatic arthritis may help improve skin psoriasis as well. Treatments for active arthritis can be more aggressive than treatments for skin disease, because joint and bone damage, unlike skin changes, are more likely to be permanent. In particular, systemic treatments are usually used for psoriatic arthritis. Some drugs being used or tested to treat both skin and joint psoriasis are methotrexate, sulfasalazine, cyclosporine, **infliximab**, **etanercept**, **adalimumab**, golimumab, and ustekinumab. These systemic treatments are usually given by either a rheumatologist or a dermatologist who specializes in psoriasis.

Diagnosis

Sacroiliac joint

The joint between the hip bones and the spine.

Oil spot

A description of the appearance of small spots (1 mm to 4 mm) on the nail in psoriasis.

Onycholysis

A medical term for nail splitting and crumbling, whether from psoriasis or another cause such as a fungus.

Infliximab

A biologic antibody therapy that works by inhibiting TNF-α, approved for the treatment of psoriasis, psoriatic arthritis, and other diseases.

Etanercept

A biologic therapy that works by inhibiting TNF-α, currently usually used to treat moderate to severe psoriasis. Sold under the trade name Enbrel.

Adalimumab

A biologic therapy that works by inhibiting TNF-α. It is currently being used and under study for the treatment of moderate to severe psoriasis.

Physicians and medical journals may use the abbreviation **PsA** or **PsoA** when referring to psoriatic arthritis, just as they may use **Ps** or **Pso** to abbreviate psoriasis.

PsA/PsoA

Abbreviation used for psoriatic arthritis.

Ps/Pso

Abbreviation used for psoriasis.

21. Is there any way to tell whether I will get psoriatic arthritis in the future?

No. At this time there is no signal that indicates whether an individual will get psoriatic arthritis in the future. No type of skin disease, blood result, or genetic test can give information that can predict whether or how psoriasis, or psoriatic arthritis, will change.

Organizations like the National Psoriasis Foundation have surveyed large numbers of people with psoriasis (more than 20,000 in the largest study) and have determined factors that seem to be associated with psoriatic arthritis in some people. In large groups of people with psoriasis, those with severe disease or with nail psoriasis were more likely than those without these changes to get psoriatic arthritis at some point in their life.

It is important to emphasize that the data on psoriatic arthritis come from studies of thousands of people and don't predict how psoriasis will behave in an individual. Although this information can suggest factors that might make a person more or less likely to develop psoriatic arthritis, each person is different. Careful observation of the skin and joints in an individual is the best way to monitor for changes in psoriasis and the development of joint disease.

22. What happens if I get psoriatic arthritis in the future?

For people who get arthritis, specific arthritis treatment may be needed to stop the disease from getting worse. For joint disease, **systemic therapy** is often needed. Some treatments for psoriasis, such as methotrexate and some biologic therapies, will treat psoriatic arthritis and skin psoriasis at the same time by decreasing inflammation throughout the body.

For people with joint disease and minimal or no skin problems, the first approach is often pain management with nonsteroidal anti-inflammatories ranging from ibuprofen (found in pain relievers such as Motrin and Advil), to prescription medications called the COX-2 inhibitors (found in medications such as Celebrex). Other oral medicines such as sulfasalazine or stronger anti-inflammatories may also be used. A rheumatologist can help decide which therapy works best for a particular person. It is important to treat this arthritis early, and to have it monitored by an expert to ensure that the therapy is working effectively. This is especially critical since joint damage can be disabling and permanent.

When a person does not have arthritis, attention to new joint pain is important. Joint pain can come from many causes, including injury or overuse. Any new joint pain should be evaluated by a physician, especially when it appears with redness, swelling, or tenderness of the surrounding tissues, or persists over time.

23. What are the different types of psoriatic arthritis?

Although there is no clear-cut set of criteria or tests for psoriatic arthritis, several distinct types have been described. The characteristic symptoms of all types of psoriatic arthritis are red hot, swollen, and tender joints. In contrast to the more common "wear and

Systemic therapy or treatment

Medications that are given in ways that make it likely that they will be absorbed throughout the body, and therefore have the potential to affect organs and systems other than the skin or joints.

The characteristic symptoms of all types of psoriatic arthritis are red hot, swollen, and tender joints.

Diagnosis

tear" of osteoarthritis, which is worse at the end of the day or after heavy use, stiffness and pain in psoriatic arthritis tend to be worse in the morning and usually last longer than 45 minutes.

Five types of psoriatic arthritis have been described; they are sometimes referred to as the Moll criteria.

Distal arthritis

Distal means far, so distal arthritis refers to arthritis at the ends of the limbs, like the hands and feet.

Oligoarthritis

Inflammation of a few (oligo-) joints (-arthritis).

Polyarthritis

A medical term referring to arthritis in many (poly-) joints (-arthritis).

Arthritis mutilans

Joint inflammation (arthritis) that causes permanent and sometimes mutilating joint changes.

Spondylarthropathy

Inflammation of the spine and hip joints.

1. **Distal arthritis** involves the small joints of the hands and feet, especially the fingers and toes.

2. **Oligoarthritis** is arthritis in which four or fewer joints are affected (oligo- means "few").

3. **Polyarthritis** is arthritis in which more than five joints are involved (poly- means "many"). This variant may appear very similar to rheumatoid arthritis.

4. **Arthritis mutilans** is a very destructive form of arthritis that may cause permanent changes in the shape of joints.

5. **Spondylarthropathy** is inflammation of the spine and hip joints.

Some people experience more than one of these types, but they all typically respond to the same treatment approaches. Early identification and appropriate treatment can help prevent worsening and possible permanent joint damage.

PART THREE

Risk, Prevention, and Epidemiology

Are there different types of psoriasis?

Will psoriasis go away?

Why do some people have mild psoriasis and others have severe disease?

More . . .

24. Are there different types of psoriasis?

Several types of psoriasis can occur on people's skin; by far the most common is plaque psoriasis, also called psoriasis vulgaris (vulgar being Latin for common). The majority of psoriasis studies focus on patients with plaque psoriasis, but most therapies will work for all types of psoriasis to some extent, as described in **Table 1**. Some people may find they have overlapping forms or a type that may evolve from one form to another over time.

John's comment:

After first being diagnosed with psoriasis some 20+ years ago, I later came to realize that when it appears on certain parts of the body it manifests in different ways. So when I would get it in different places, sometimes I didn't realize it was psoriasis until the dermatologist would say "yes, that is also psoriasis."

Human leukocyte antigen (HLA) system

Proteins located on the surface of white blood cells that play an important role in our body's immune response to foreign substances.

Chromosome

A molecule of DNA found in the nucleus of every cell, chromosomes contain the cell's genetic information. Humans normally have 46 chromosomes.

25. Is psoriasis genetic? Will I give it to my children, or will I get it if a relative has the disease?

Psoriasis is thought to be caused by a combination of genetics and environment. Although several genes have been associated with an increased risk of psoriasis, the significance of any one gene in the development of psoriasis is not known.

Several genes are more common in psoriasis sufferers and less common in the general population. Although the genes have many different functions, most are part of the immune system. The most important ones are part of the HLA, or **human leukocyte antigen (HLA) system**. The HLA is a group of genes on **chromosome** 6

Table 1 Treatments for Different Forms of Psoriasis

Type	Approximate % of Patients	Body Areas	Commonly Affects	Type-Specific Signs or Symptoms	Common Treatments	Treatment Challenges	Comments
Plaque (vulgaris)	85%	Elbows, knees, trunk, legs	Adults	Red, scaly thickened areas that may be quite large	Topical steroids, vitamin A and D derivatives, light; systemic therapies for moderate and severe disease	When large body surface areas are affected, a lot of topical products may be required	Most common form studied in clinical trials
Scalp psoriasis	50% or more	Scalp, often asymmetric distribution	Adults, children	Scale usually predominates over redness and thickness on scalp	Topical steroids, tar, and vitamin D derivatives in scalp formulations such as solution or foam; scalp oils; keratolytics to loosen scale	Most creams and ointments are difficult to apply to hair-bearing skin	May overlap with seborrheic dermatitis and respond to antifungals; avoid picking or scratching scalp as it may worsen the disease through Koebnerization

Continued

Table 1   Treatments for Different Forms of Psoriasis (continued)

Type	Approximate % of Patients	Body Areas	Commonly Affects	Type-Specific Signs or Symptoms	Common Treatments	Treatment Challenges	Comments
Palmar-plantar	3% to 4%	Hands and feet	Adults	May appear scaly and hyperkeratotic, or as pustules, or both	Super-potent topical steroids, vitamin A derivatives, tar; local phototherapy to hands and feet; therapy under occlusion, such as tape; systemic therapies; avoid irritation like harsh soaps and frequent washing	Thick skin of palms and soles impedes penetration of medication; frequent hand washing and hand trauma are difficult to avoid and may worsen condition	Therapy under occlusion can be accomplished by applying medication, then wearing cotton gloves and socks overnight; local PUVA can be helpful
Inverse	3% to 4%	Primarily armpits, groin, inside of elbows and knees	Adults	In men, in groin or "jock itch" area; in women, in skin folds under breasts	Mild to moderate topical steroids; topical immunomodulators like tacrolimus and pimecrolimus; antifungals if a fungal infection is also present	Thin skin of skin folds is very sensitive to side effects of topical steroids; can be hard to treat	Avoid irritating underarm deodorants, tight clothes; cotton undergarments can be helpful
Guttate	Less than 20%, increased in children	All over body	More common in children and young adults	Known to follow a streptococcal throat infection	UV light, topicals, sometimes systemic therapies; antibiotics to treat infection if needed	May recur if infection returns	Other triggers include viral infections, medications

Pustular	Less than 2%	Usually all over body or hands and feet	Adults	Often seen as a flare after a triggering event or with rapid withdrawal of all therapy	Oral retinoids, cyclosporine, methotrexate, phototherapy, biologics may be useful	Can be very uncomfortable and difficult to treat	May be seen when tapering oral steroids
Erythro-dermic	Less than 4%	Whole body	Adults	May develop after stress such as withdrawal after a course of oral steroids or after a phototherapy burn	Severe disease, though rare, may require hospitalization; systemic therapy usually prescribed	Important for a physician to distinguish it from other causes of erythroderma (red skin covering the body); risk of infection of the blood	More common historically; reduced incidence now with more effective and aggressive treatments
Psoriatic arthritis	5% to 30%	Several patterns of joint involvement	More common in people with psoriasis on the nails and people with more severe psoriasis	Commonly affects finger joints and lower back	Anti-inflammatories to treat joint pain; systemic therapies that can slow or stop joint damage	May require systemic treatment, which may need to be continuous; rheumatologist may help determine what to use	Joint changes may be permanent

(continued)

Table 1 Treatments for Different Forms of Psoriasis (continued)

Type	Approximate % of Patients	Body Areas	Commonly Affects	Type-Specific Signs or Symptoms	Common Treatments	Treatment Challenges	Comments
Nail psoriasis	Up to 75%	Both fingers and toes	People with more severe disease, people with psoriatic arthritis	Psoriasis spots occur at points under the nail bed, and the nail separates from the bed, creating spots	Wrapping nails with steroid-containing tape, steroid cream under tape or plastic wrap, steroid injection into nail beds	Topically applied steroids typically do not penetrate well into the nail bed for effective therapy	Wearing shoes with a wide toe box can prevent further nail disfiguration; systemic treatments for skin or joint disease will often treat the nails, also
Genital psoriasis	3% to 4%	Groin; may affect head of penis or vulva	Adults, babies	Redness is more common than flaky scale on genital skin	Low potency topical steroids, immuno-modulators such as tacrolimus and pimecrolimus	Thin skin of treatment areas increases risks of side effects; avoid potent and super-potent topical steroids	

that encodes sequences, or directions, for proteins on white blood cells. The white blood cells, primed to defend against infection, are sometimes activated inappropriately. In psoriasis and other immune-mediated diseases, the immune system, led by the white blood cells, is inappropriately activated in different parts of the body. In psoriasis, these white cells, including a subset called T cells, become activated in areas of skin. These areas of skin respond with the skin thickening, redness, and the scale of psoriasis.

Efforts to scan the entire genome of psoriasis patients have confirmed that there are multiple common genes associated with psoriasis. These reports continue to show that HLA-C is of substantial importance and also implicate genes related to interleukin 12, interleukin 23, and tumor necrosis factor (TNF). These discoveries are consistent with our knowledge about how some of the newer biologic therapies are known to work. (See Questions 65 and 66.) Affected people may have a combination of several relevant genetic variants that predisposes them to the disease.

At this time, the interaction between these genes, the T cells that carry them, and changes in the skin are still being explored. The knowledge we have, however, provides hope that there may be improved therapy in the future based on a person's genetics. These results are still preliminary and currently cannot be used to determine the risk of psoriasis, disease prognosis, or therapy. No genetic tests are available or required to treat psoriasis.

Although psoriasis has a genetic component, it is not a predictably inherited disease. When a person has psoriasis, the chance of his or her child acquiring the disease is less than 20%. There is no blood test, genetic

In psoriasis and other immune-mediated diseases, the immune system, led by the white blood cells, is inappropriately activated in different parts of the body.

test, or prenatal diagnostic that currently predicts whether a baby will have psoriasis in the future. This means that when one family member has psoriasis, the risk is increased for the other family members but cannot be predicted for a specific person.

Studies have guided our understanding of genetics in psoriasis, but can be limited by the availability of information on family members. For example, psoriasis might be described by some as "bad dandruff" or eczema, depending on how it appears. As a result, the exact chance of a person getting psoriasis can be hard to predict.

26. Does psoriasis tend to be stable or does it fluctuate over time?

Psoriasis does not have a predictable course, so it is impossible to predict whether a particular person will improve or worsen over time. For people with known triggers that exacerbate their disease, exposure to these factors, such as stress, may predict worsening, while reduction of these triggers could predict stabilization or improvement.

In a study of 5,600 patients conducted at Stanford University in 1974, slightly over half the people had experienced at least one period of time when their psoriasis was completely healed (in remission). In this group, the remission period lasted an average of 5 months. (For the purposes of this study, remission was defined as an absence of psoriasis without treatment.) Of those people, over 95% saw their psoriasis return within 6 months to 2 years.

Over time, a person's psoriasis can behave in different ways, but people appear to adapt more easily to these changes after years with the disease. Sufferers may find that flares or changes are easier to deal with after they've identified effective treatments and routines for their skin.

27. Why do some people have mild psoriasis and others have severe disease?

It's not known why one person has a mild form of psoriasis and another a severe form or why one person has nail changes while another does not. Over time, psoriasis severity and location may change and evolve or get better or worse. Unfortunately, more is known about what makes psoriasis get worse than what makes it get better. Strangely, the severity of psoriatic arthritis and the severity of skin psoriasis often do not correspond.

Research thus far shows that the degree of treatment, whether very aggressive or none at all, does not alter the course or severity of the disease. Early onset of psoriasis, in the early 20s or before, is more strongly linked to a family history and is more likely to become severe over time.

Early onset of psoriasis, in the early 20s or before, is more strongly linked to a family history and is more likely to become severe over time.

In the large study at Stanford University described in Question 26, almost 40% of people experienced disease-free periods of over 1 year. These statistics may have improved in the subsequent 30 years because of the many new therapies developed since then.

28. Will psoriasis go away?

For some people, their psoriasis may disappear for a period of time. For others, this may never occur. Generally, people with mild psoriasis—less than 5% of

Body surface area (BSA)

The area of skin on a person, measured in square feet or square meters. Usually used as a percentage to describe the proportion of the body's skin that is affected or covered.

their **body surface area (BSA)** affected, or "just a few spots"—are more likely to experience a remission than people with more extensive disease. It is important to note that while psoriasis may disappear, there is no specific treatment that will put it into permanent remission or cure it at this time.

It is very difficult to predict how psoriasis will act in the future for any one person. Some people may recall circumstances where their psoriasis was at its "best" or least severe or even resolved. If people can associate disease resolution with decreased stress, such as a vacation, or with more sunlight, such as living in a sunny location, it may predict for them which circumstances are most likely to decrease psoriasis.

The possibility of making psoriasis go away is a very appealing one, and many current treatments may suggest they can provide this effect. Although a product may make psoriasis go away in one person, its effect on a given person can't be predicted. Claims to make psoriasis "go away" need to be appraised with a critical eye. At this point, a cure is not known.

29. Will eating or avoiding certain foods help my psoriasis?

There is not one universal diet that has been shown to make psoriasis predictably better or worse. However, many individuals report that a link exists for them between psoriasis severity and diet. Many people will try different diets and, over time, find one that works well for them. Psoriasis sufferers have reported the associations listed in **Table 2** and many others probably exist.

Of the supplements listed in Table 2, several studies on fish oil have been formally reported. Some small studies

Table 2   Association of Foods and Supplements with Psoriasis

	Reported to Help Psoriasis	Reported to Worsen Psoriasis
Foods	Fish	Gluten (a component of wheat) Milk
Supplements	Vitamins: zinc, folate, iron Fish oil Tumeric Flax seed oil Milk thistle Oregano oil Shark cartilage	

have shown improvement when fish oil was given orally or by vein. One study showed that oral fish oil worked better than olive oil when given with light therapy. Another study from the same group showed that fish oil was not better than olive oil when used in combination with topical steroids. A much larger study, published in 1993, showed fish oil was no better than corn oil. Although associations between these supplements and skin improvement have been reported, for some, no response or even an opposite response may be seen. It is useful to discover what works best for your psoriasis through trial and error.

If a person is interested in making a diet change, making one change at a time will help to identify exacerbating or helpful diet changes. When making a diet change, make sure to give it at least 2 to 4 weeks before coming to a conclusion. Psoriasis may wax and wane over time independently of diet as well. Knowing that other external factors, such as stress and sunlight (see Question 93), may affect psoriasis, it is worth considering possible effects of these changes when evaluating a diet or any new therapy.

Because of a possible association of psoriasis and celiac disease (sensitivity to wheat gluten), many people with psoriasis have tried a gluten-free diet. Gluten is the insoluble component of grains such as wheat, barley, and rye, and people with celiac disease have an immuno-logic reaction to gluten. However, this diet is a very challenging one and a trial of weeks to months is often recommended. If a person has gastrointestinal symp-toms like bloating, diarrhea, or abdominal pain, evalu-ation with a physician including possible blood tests for celiac disease could be considered.

One excellent resource to learn about people's individ-ual experiences is a feature from the National Psoriasis Foundation's bimonthly magazine called "It Works For Me." Previous submissions are archived on their Web site (more information is in the Appendix). In these testimonials, people with psoriasis and psoriatic arthri-tis share treatments they have found effective, from medicines to foods to exercise regimens and more.

30. I have psoriasis in the area of an old scar. Is this common? Why is this?

Psoriasis very often appears where skin has previously been injured. This phenomenon is called the Koebner phenomenon. It is named after its discoverer, Dr. Heinrich Koebner, a dermatologist in Germany who first described the phenomenon in 1872. The appear-ance of psoriasis after trauma is often called Koebner-ization and usually appears between 2 and 6 weeks after trauma to the skin. This phenomenon is found in some people with psoriasis, as well as those with other skin diseases like vitiligo and warts.

Koebnerization is thought to occur through the normal inflammation in traumatized skin. When skin is injured, a normal inflammatory reaction occurs with redness, warmth, pain, and swelling. In normal skin this inflammation resolves after the skin damage is healed. In contrast, the inflammatory reaction in a psoriatic patient attracts the skin-reactive immune cells in addition to the normal response. These cells don't simply aid in skin repair, but create changes in psoriasis in the traumatized area.

One reason that psoriasis is thought to be common on the elbows and knees is that these locations are constantly exposed to the slight trauma of stretching at flexible joints and rubbing against hard surfaces, which may cause ongoing Koebnerization at these sites.

Because of the Koebner phenomenon, traumatic skin procedures should be avoided whenever possible. Tattoos, including permanent makeup, can cause trauma that leads to Koebnerization. Skin-resurfacing techniques such as dermabrasion, often used for acne scars and skin tightening, could cause Koebnerization and psoriatic changes in previously healthy facial skin.

When trauma does occur, protect the skin as much as possible with occlusive bandages such as Band-Aids or other wound dressings. Keep injured skin greasy with ointments such as Aquaphor or Vaseline, or antibiotic ointments such as bacitracin, mupirocin (Bactroban), neomycin (Neosporin), or polymyxin (in Polysporin). Contrary to popular belief it is not necessary for a scab to form in order for the skin to heal. In fact, the presence of a hard scab can block the skin from covering an injured area. Avoid drying out injured areas since dryness can cause skin tightness, scab formation, and rebreaking of the skin. Strong antiseptics like hydrogen peroxide or rubbing alcohol are rarely needed. Diligent care for skin injuries can minimize or prevent Koebnerization of psoriasis to injured skin.

The potential for Koebnerization varies among people, and not every person will have problems with psoriasis appearing after trauma. For unknown reasons, this phenomenon can come and go over a lifetime.

For unknown reasons, this phenomenon can come and go over a lifetime.

31. I was diagnosed with pustular psoriasis. Do I have an infection?

Although the word "pustular" conjures the image of an infection or abscess, pustular psoriasis is not an infection. The pustular name describes the skin's appearance, where yellow pus is seen scattered in blister-like areas beneath the surface of psoriatic skin. These pustules are sometimes referred to as "sterile pustules," meaning that they are free of any bacteria or infection. The presence of pus and yellow color is due to the presence of a type of white blood cell called a neutrophil, which usually attacks bacteria. In this situation, the neutrophils are being recruited to psoriatic skin without an infection, and instead of responding to infection, they form blisters full of pus.

Superinfection

An infection that develops following another skin problem, such as psoriasis or eczema, for example. This infection is often more persistent or more difficult to treat than an infection on previously healthy skin.

Pustular psoriasis is not an infection, but it is possible for people with psoriasis to have infections of the skin at the same time. When people have psoriasis, it is possible to have a **superinfection**, meaning an infection that occurs at the same location of another skin disease, including psoriasis. If one or two pustules occur on skin with psoriasis, and the area feels warm, swollen, or painful, it suggests that the pustules may be caused by an infection rather than the psoriasis alone.

Most of the medicines used to treat more common forms of psoriasis have also been used successfully to treat pustular psoriasis. Acitretin (sold as Soriatane), alone or in combination with other therapies, is chosen frequently as a treatment for this kind of psoriasis.

Pustular psoriasis can be associated with fever, chills, or abnormalities in blood chemistry. If pustules appear on the body, physician attention should be sought immediately.

32. Can babies get psoriasis?

It is very unusual for a baby to get psoriasis, but it does occur. Most often, the condition starts as a red rash in the diaper area that doesn't clear up with typical diaper rash treatments. It might appear somewhat different than diaper rash, but it may take an experienced pediatric dermatologist to tell the difference between psoriasis, seborrheic dermatitis (cradle cap), and diaper rash in some children.

If a baby has what looks like a diaper rash, it is most probably just that, even if a parent or family member has psoriasis. Although babies can get psoriasis, the great majority of all babies, with or without a family history of psoriasis, will experience diaper rash from normal causes. Unlike the usual course of events in adults, when children do get psoriasis, it may resolve completely and never return.

33. Do children get psoriasis, and does it go away?

Yes, children can get psoriasis. Although psoriasis is less common in children, and may appear differently than in adults, children can get psoriasis. Among adults with psoriasis, 30% to 45% had the onset of their disease before age 20. Psoriasis is slightly more common in boys than in girls, and almost 70% of children who get psoriasis have family members with psoriasis. For reasons that are unclear, psoriasis often first appears in the fall.

Although children and young adults may get any type of psoriasis, one type found almost exclusively in children or younger patients and young adults is guttate psoriasis (see color plate C). Guttate is Latin for raindrop and describes the small, 0.25- to 0.5-inch (0.64- to 1.3- cm) psoriasis spots that are scattered over the body like raindrops.

Unlike other types of psoriasis, guttate psoriasis is often associated with an infection and resolves when the infection goes away. An infection causes an overactive immune reaction, where T cells become activated in the skin in different spots in addition to the infection. In children, the most common infections are pharyngitis (infection of the throat), dermatitis (skin infection), and ear infections. A pediatrician or pediatric dermatologist, after recognizing the infection, will look for the infectious source and begin treatment with antibiotics. If antibiotics treat the infection properly, the skin lesions can resolve in weeks or months. If the infection returns, or a new infection develops, the guttate psoriasis may return and can be treated the same way.

Fortunately, guttate psoriasis is not always associated with the chronic plaque-type form usually seen in adults. A childhood episode has not been proven to increase or decrease the lifetime risk of acquiring common adult forms of psoriasis. However, a study conclusively proving or disproving a relationship has not yet been done.

In addition to guttate psoriasis seen after strep infection, children can get all forms of psoriasis. In children, psoriasis is often confused with diaper rash, eczema, a yeast infection, or cradle-cap (seborrheic dermatitis). Over time, the diagnosis can usually be made by the skin's appearance, and in most cases a skin biopsy is not needed.

In children, psoriasis affects the scalp about half the time. Children who get psoriasis are more likely than adults to have psoriasis on the face and on the nails.

Treatment options for children are the same as those for adults, but greater care must be taken to minimize side effects. Particularly when using topical medications, the degree of **systemic absorption** can be higher in children. In general, children should avoid using super-potent topical steroids (Class I or II; see **Table 3**), especially over long periods of time. Treatment considerations are sometimes different than in adults because the side effects of some medications in a growing child may be different than in older people.

Systemic absorption
The absorption of a medication through the skin, for example, into the blood where it reaches the entire body.

Challenges particular to children and teens with psoriasis often revolve around appearance issues and consistent use of treatment. Resources such as the National Psoriasis Foundation have dedicated message boards and online chat rooms for children, teens, and their parents to interact with other people with psoriasis.

Treatment options for children are the same as those for adults, but greater care must be taken to minimize side effects.

Table 3 Class of Topical Steroids

Class	Active Ingredient Name	Brand Name	Available Formulations
Class I: super-potent	Clobetasol propionate	Temovate, Olux	Cream, ointment, foam
	Halobetasol propionate	Ultravate	Ointment
	Betamethasone dipropionate	Diprolene	Cream, ointment
	Diflorasone diacetate	Psorcon	Ointment
Class II: potent	Amcinonide	Cyclocort	Ointment
	Betamethasone dipropionate	Diprolene	Cream AF
	Mometasone furoate	Elocon	Ointment
	Diflorasone diacetate	Florone	Ointment
	Halocinide	Halog	Cream
	Fluocinonide	Lidex	Cream, gel, ointment
	Diflorasone diacetate	Maxiflor	Ointment
	Desoximethasone	Topicort	Ointment, cream, gel
Class III: potent	Triamcinalone acetonide	Aristocort A	0.1% ointment
	Fluticasone propionate	Cutivate	Ointment
	Amcinonide	Cyclocort	Cream, solution
	Betamethasone dipropionate	Diprosone	Cream
	Diflorasone diacetate	Florone, Maxiflor	Cream
	Halocinonide	Halog	Ointment
	Fluocinonide	Lidex E	Emollient cream
	Betamethasone valerate	Valisone	Ointment

Class IV: mid-strength	Clocortolone pivalate	Cloderm	Cream
	Flurandrenolide	Cordran	Ointment, tape
	Prednicarbate	Dermatop	Ointment
	Monometasone furoate	Elocon	Cream
	Triamcinolone acetonide	Kenalog	0.5% cream, aerosol, suspension for injection
	Hydrocortisone probutate	Pandel	Cream
	Fluocinolone acetonide	Synalar	Ointment
	Hydrocortisone valerate	Westcort	Ointment
Class V: mid-strength	Flurandrenolide	Cordran	Cream
	Fluticasone propionate	Cutivate	Cream
	Prednicarbate	Dermatop	Cream
	Betamethasone dipropionate	Diprosone	Solution
	Triamcinalone acetonide	Kenalog	Solution, 0.1% cream
	Hydrocortisone butyrate	Locoid	Cream, ointment, solution
	Betamethasone valerate	Luxiq	Foam
	Fluocinolone acetate	Synalar	Cream
	Betamethasone valerate	Beta-val	Cream
	Hydrocortisone valerate	Westcort	Cream
Class VI: mild	Alclomethasone dipropionate	Aclovate	Cream, ointment
	Triamcinolone acetonide	Aristocort A	0.025% cream
	Desonide	Desowen, Trideslon	Cream, lotion, ointment
	Fluocinolone acetonide	Synalar	Ointment, cream, solution
	Betamethasone valerate	Valisone	Solution
Class VII: mild, over the counter, and by prescription	Hydrocortisone	Many brand names	Multiple formulas and sizes
	Hydrocortisone acetate	Many brand names	

Classification of the steroids into potency groups can vary from source to source, but generally does not differ by more than one group.

57

PART FOUR

Treatment

What options do I have to treat my psoriasis,
and do I need to treat it to keep it
from getting worse?

Are there different treatments for different kinds
of psoriasis?

Does health insurance cover psoriasis
treatment?

More . . .

34. What options do I have to treat my psoriasis, and do I need to treat it to keep it from getting worse?

There are many different treatments for psoriasis. Some may work better than others for a particular person, and their effectiveness may change over time. For these reasons, it can be helpful to be aware of all available options.

Broadly, treatments can be based by formula (how they're given) or type (how they work).

By formula:

- Topical medications
- Ointment: Medication in an oil-based **vehicle** (e.g. Vaseline and Aquaphor)
- Cream: Usually medication in a **base** made of water mixed with oil
- **Solution**: Medication in water or water mixed with alcohol, sometimes called a **lotion**
- **Foam**: Medication in an alcohol-based or water-based foam (consistency similar to hair mousse)
- Tape: Medication in an adhesive tape that sticks to the skin
- Gel: Medication in an alcohol or water-based formulation with a thick consistency (similar to hair gel)
- Spray: Medication in water and/or alcohol that is aerosolized into tiny droplets applied to the skin as a mist
- Oral medications
- Injectable medications
- Subcutaneous: Under the skin
- Intramuscular: Into a muscle
- Intravenous: Into a vein
- Ultraviolet light sources

Vehicle
The base or inactive product into which a medication is mixed. Examples include petrolatum, cream, and foam.

Base
The type of substance that a topical medicine may be formulated in (an ointment, cream, lotion, or foam).

Solution
A mixture of a medicine in water, or water with alcohol, for topical use, often on hair-bearing areas. Sometimes referred to as a "lotion."

Lotion
A water-based, or water-and alcohol-based, topical medication used to treat the skin, sometimes called a "solution."

Foam
An inert base or vehicle made of alcohol and/or water in which an active ingredient such as a topical steroid can be mixed. A foam may appear similar in consistency to hair mousse but is used on the skin.

- Full-body light box
- Hands- or feet-only light box
- Natural sunlight
- Hand-held light units
- Lasers

By type:

- Steroid-based medications: Topical steroids, steroid injections into local areas, steroid tape
- Vitamin D analogs: **Calcipotriene** or **calcipotriol** (two names for the same medication) and **calcitriol**. There is also a combination ointment that contains calcipotriene and the steroid betamethasone.
- Vitamin A analogs: **Tazarotene, acitretin**
- UV radiation and light-based therapies: UVB, PUVA, **narrow-band UVB**, tanning beds, lasers (**excimer laser**), natural sunlight
- Nonsteroid immunosuppressants: Cyclosporine, **tacrolimus** (oral and topical), **pimecrolimus** (topical only), and sulfasalazine
- Drugs that affect cell metabolism: Methotrexate, mycophenolate mofetil, and hydroxyurea
- Biologic therapies: Infliximab, etanercept, **alefacept**, adalimumab, ustekinumab, and golimumab

The choice of treatments might be based on a variety of factors, including:

- Effectiveness
- Safety
- Convenience
- Facilities available in your area; light therapy and "day care" may require travel
- Medicine preferences, such as topical medications vs. oral

Treatment

Calcipotriene (calcipotriol)

A topically applied vitamin D derivative used to treat psoriasis.

Calcitriol

A topically applied vitamin D derivative used to treat psoriasis.

Tazarotene

A topical vitamin A derivative developed to treat psoriasis. An oral form is in development.

Acitretin

A vitamin A derivative taken by mouth usually used to treat moderate to severe psoriasis.

Narrow-band UVB

Narrow-band UVB refers to a specific wavelength of UV radiation (311 to 313 nm). This range has proven the most beneficial component of natural sunlight for psoriasis.

Excimer laser

A laser used by dermatologists that works at 311-nm wavelength, similar to the wavelength of UVB. It has been effective for treating psoriasis in local areas and is given in a dermatologist's office.

How psoriasis responds when treatment is stopped depends on the person's underlying disease and which treat-ments they have been using.

- Other diseases you may have
- Other medications you are taking
- Whether you have arthritis with your psoriasis
- Insurance coverage of different therapies

The initial choice of treatment can be made with these issues in mind, and most people continue to change or adjust their psoriasis medication over time. It is impor-tant to know the various options available and to con-sider a different approach if a regimen loses its effectiveness.

Finally, it is not absolutely necessary to treat psoriasis, especially if very mild. Some people become concerned that psoriasis, if not treated aggressively, will continue to worsen. This isn't necessarily true. How psoriasis responds when treatment is stopped depends on the person's underlying disease and which treatments they have been using.

35. How can I decide which treatment is best for me?

Harold's comment:

Work with your doctor and start with the mildest treatment—one that's easy to adhere to and that you will follow religiously. Keep adjusting the treatment until you see positive results.

Treatment of psoriasis is always individualized for a particular person. Partnership with a dermatologist, a family practitioner, or other healing individual can help to develop a plan for long-term therapy. Many people find that a physician experienced in treating psoriasis is especially helpful. Therapy that works well for one person might not be effective for another, and fine-tuning or changing medication is often required.

The initial choice of medication will depend on psoriasis severity, its location, and the preferences of a particular patient. For mild, moderate, and some severe disease, **topical treatments** are usually tried first and are generally effective. Certain situations, such as the presence of arthritis, psoriasis on the hands and feet, drug allergies, pregnancy, or medications taken for other conditions, will influence the initial choice of therapy.

Almost all therapies require consistent use in order to be effective, and most take a continuous 6- to 8-week trial to find out whether they are working. When using any medication, it is important to use it consistently and continuously so that it becomes clear whether a particular medication is effective.

Some physicians utilize specialized treatment strategies by rotating, combining, or sequencing different therapies for an individual (discussed in Question 62). Over time, individuals can identify which therapies or combinations are most effective for their skin and most convenient for their lifestyles.

36. Are there different treatments for different kinds of psoriasis?

Because all types of psoriasis have the same underlying cause, all psoriasis treatments will work to some extent for most types of psoriasis. There are, however, a few treatment approaches that can maximize the effectiveness of therapies in different types of psoriasis.

Topical treatment
A treatment administered on the skin to treat an infection locally.

Treatment

- Plaque psoriasis: All prescription psoriasis treatments have been proven to treat this most common type of psoriasis. Because most treatments are effective, people may consider rotating different medicines and trying different formulas to find the right one for them.

- Palmar-plantar psoriasis: Although topical medicines are effective, they may need more time or more frequent use to penetrate through the thick skin of hands and feet. Ointments, frequent application, or use under **occlusion** at night (using plastic wrap or cotton socks and gloves) can maximize the effectiveness of topical medications. Systemic treatments aren't always indicated for palmar-plantar psoriasis, but when overall disease is severe and disabling, some people experience good improvement with more aggressive treatment such as topical PUVA or **systemic medications**. Retinoids such as acitretin are often used in this scenario.

- Scalp psoriasis: Medications in solution or foam formulations penetrate scalp skin well, while leaving the least amount of medication on the hair. In addition to using psoriasis medicines, specific treatments to loosen scale can be very effective. In particular, **keratolytics** (compounds that break up scale), anti-dandruff shampoos, and oils are effective for many people.

- Inverse and genital psoriasis: Although the same topical treatments are effective, thin skin in the skin folds (under the arm pits, around the groin, and under a woman's breasts) and on the genitals requires special attention. In particular, this thin and sometimes sensitive skin absorbs medication very rapidly and is more susceptible to both the therapeutic effects

Occlusion

Covering, for example, with cotton (cotton socks or gloves), plastic wrap, or tape.

Systemic medication

A medication given, either by mouth or by injection, to reach the entire body.

Keratolytic

A compound that helps remove dead skin cells from the epidermis and breaks down keratin in scale. One example is the group of alpha hydroxy acids.

and unwanted side effects of topical medications. For this reason, milder steroids (Class V or below) should be used in these areas. Certain topical **immunomodulators**, called tacrolimus and pimecrolimus, can be effective on the skin folds and genitals as well. These medications show modest benefit for "regular" plaque psoriasis but are more effective (and with minimal side effects) in sensitive skin areas.

- Nail psoriasis: The nail changes of psoriasis are particularly challenging to treat for two reasons. First, it is very difficult to get medication to reach the nail bed where new, healthy nail is growing. Second, nails grow slowly, so any treatment takes a long time to take effect. Choices include topical therapies that penetrate well (strong steroids under occlusion, for example), steroid injections into the base of the nail behind the cuticle, and systemic treatments for those who have more severe overall disease.

37. Does health insurance cover psoriasis treatment?

Although each insurance plan is different, medical insurance, including **Medicare**, normally covers the cost of physician visits to treat psoriasis. **Prescription drugs**, depending on the details of a particular plan, are covered by most commercial insurance plans. When a medication is covered, typically the costs of side-effect monitoring for that medication (with blood tests, for example) are covered as well.

Other therapies, such as the newer biologics in use, may be covered only after other therapies have failed or if you have psoriatic arthritis as well as psoriasis.

Immunomodulator

A medication that modifies how the immune system functions or responds.

Medicare

The primary health insurance program for people over the age of 65 and those with certain disabilities. Medicare provides for acute hospital care, physician services, short stays in nursing facilities, and short-term home care for a medical problem. Coverage is restricted to medical care, to prescription drugs under certain limits, though not custodial care at home or in a nursing home. It was established by Congress in 1935.

Prescription drug

A drug available only by the prescription of a physician. These drugs have been formally tested and are regulated by the FDA.

Your employer, insurance company, or physician will have more information about the details of a particular health plan. Some systemic treatments, such as the newer biologic therapies, require **preauthorization** or prior permission from an insurance company before being used. Some insurance companies require evidence that other systemic therapies such as cyclosporine or methotrexate are ineffective before giving authorization for treatments. Some plans require a letter of medical necessity from a treating physician. Sample letters to insurance plans can be found at the National Psoriasis Foundation Web site, and many drug manufacturers have specialized groups that help physicians and patients navigate through the approval process (see Appendix for more information).

Preauthorization

Pretreatment clearance from an insurance company to use a particular therapy. The process usually involves a physician corresponding with an insurance company on a patient's behalf.

What is not covered by insurance is the cost of any medicine available over-the-counter at the drugstore. This includes nonprescription drugs such as Benadryl (diphenhydramine), nonprescription lotions or creams, nonprescription shampoos, and nonprescription medicated creams such as hydrocortisone or Sarna. People with psoriasis may use a significant amount of cream and other skin care products, and the cost of treatment is a common challenge for many psoriasis sufferers.

One of the many challenging aspects of psoriasis is its constant and often high cost of treatment.

One of the many challenging aspects of psoriasis is its constant and often high cost of treatment. Research has confirmed that higher out-of-pocket costs add to the suffering of people with psoriasis and other skin diseases.

Jason's comment:

Just because your insurer's first answer is "no" doesn't mean that's the final word. Ask for individual consideration, and ask your dermatologist to help.

38. How do I select a dermatologist?

Harold's comment:

Ask around; more people have psoriasis than you think. If that doesn't work, go online and do some research.

Consider some or all of the following factors when choosing a dermatologist:

• Insurance coverage: Does a physician accept a particular health plan?
• Location and hours of clinic: Is it convenient to make appointments?
• Availability of physician: How soon can I get an appointment?
• Physician's background and training: Do they have experience treating psoriasis?
• Recommendations from friends, family, or colleagues
• Recommendations from other people with psoriasis

Different physicians specialize within the field of dermatology. A physician's practice may focus on **medical dermatology**, treating skin diseases such as psoriasis. These dermatologists are usually the most experienced in treating psoriasis and have the most experience trying different therapies for challenging cases. Other dermatologists may focus on children's dermatology, dermatologic surgery, cosmetic dermatology, or dermatopathology. With this in mind, it may be helpful to inquire whether a physician treats many people with psoriasis.

Medical dermatology

The branch of dermatology that treats medical diseases of the skin, such as psoriasis, that may need systemic drug therapy, or skin changes that arise from systemic diseases.

Two resources for finding dermatologists in your area include the American Academy of Dermatology and the National Psoriasis Foundation (see Appendix).

39. What should I ask my dermatologist?

If you have recently been diagnosed with psoriasis, you probably have many questions about the disease and its treatment. When meeting a dermatologist for the first time, it can be helpful to write down specific questions you would like answered. Make sure, however, that you give your doctor time to talk about what he or she thinks, too. Sometimes all your questions will be answered in the process—and you may learn about some other important points and tips along the way.

Over time, the appearance of psoriasis may change or your treatment preferences may change. Some people may tire of using time-consuming topical medicines, whereas others may become concerned about the potential side effects of a treatment over the long term. You might wonder, "What are some other treatments I can use for my skin?" The psoriasis armamentarium contains many medications, and a physician should be able to help you select different treatments over time.

When considering a new medication, be sure to review the following with your doctor:

- How do I use this properly? Consider medication amount, schedule, and how to apply or take a medicine. For example, some oral medications should be taken with food, and some topical medications should be applied in a certain way. (For example, foam can melt, so it may be helpful to spray it into the cap and apply it from there rather than your hand.)
- What side effects should I look for? Some topical medications may cause itching or burning, and some oral medications may affect your energy level. Knowing what to expect can help you get used to different side effects.

- What are the signs that I should stop the medication? Review which side effects usually improve over time and which indicate that the medication should be stopped.
- When should I expect to see improvements? Some medications take days to work and others may take weeks to months.
- When should I return? Most physicians will tell you when to return, and it can be useful to make a plan for the frequency of visits. Make sure you understand what factors (abnormal blood tests, new side effects, worsening psoriasis) indicate that it is time to see a physician.

40. Should I get a second opinion on my diagnosis or treatment?

Because psoriasis is usually a clinical diagnosis, you might wonder if the diagnosis is accurate. For the majority of people with the most common or classic signs of psoriasis, the diagnosis is straightforward, and a second opinion will not add new information.

If the symptoms of someone's skin disease are not consistent with psoriasis in terms of location (discussed in Question 8) or appearance, it is sometimes referred to as an **atypical presentation** of the disease. In this situation, some physicians may order a skin biopsy, while others may begin with treatment to see if the skin improves. A skin biopsy can be helpful to establish a diagnosis, but will leave a small but permanent scar on the skin. Both approaches are common.

A second opinion can be useful if the psoriasis looks atypical or does not respond to treatment. Similarly, if psoriasis worsens dramatically, a different physician

Atypical presentation

A situation in which a disease arises and appears different than normal (in a different place or with a different appearance, for example), usually necessitating further tests for an accurate diagnosis.

may be able to suggest other treatment options. The cost of a second opinion visit may or may not be covered by insurance, so it may be worthwhile to call your insurance plan if you plan to seek a second opinion.

While you may hear different information from varying sources such as family, friends, an internist, or a dermatologist, it is important that you feel as comfortable as possible with your diagnosis and treatment plan. This may include seeking the expertise and care of a different physician.

41. What if I don't like my doctor?

The decision to change doctors is a personal one based on your experiences and further questions you may have. You might wish to change physicians when a physician cannot suggest further treatment options or if you feel that communication with your physician is not effective.

Several resources exist for finding a physician expert in psoriasis, including the National Psoriasis Foundation, the American Academy of Dermatology, the dermatology department or division at a medical school in your area, and recommendations from other people with psoriasis. Your dermatologist or medical doctor may be able to recommend a psoriasis expert nearby. As a starting point, most of this information can be found on the Internet.

To get the most out of a new appointment, carefully select a knowledgeable physician ahead of time.

To get the most out of a new appointment, carefully select a knowledgeable physician ahead of time. Gather all your current medications for psoriasis and other diseases. Record all prior medications used to treat psoriasis. Particularly for oral medications, dosages and periods of time used are required to help evaluate the risk of side effects. Ask your current doctor to give you copies of clinic notes, laboratory work, and a pathology report if a biopsy was done. Gathering this information ahead of time makes a consultation more effective and helps to avoid a delay in sending records between offices. Bring the name and address of a physician who knows you (another dermatologist, your internist, or another physician you see regularly), and the results of your appointment will be reported in a letter from the new consultant to your regular doctor. Recognize that it may take more than one visit to get all of your questions answered and that forming a working relationship over time is a critical part of your care.

At the end of a new consultation, you have the opportunity to return to your treating physician or to continue care with the consulting physician. Factors such as personal preferences, convenience, availability, or coverage by a particular insurance plan may be important factors in that decision. Whoever you decide to use as your primary physician for psoriasis, it is important to stay in close contact with him or her to coordinate your care, watch for medication side effects over time, monitor blood work if needed, and be the primary individual responsible for monitoring your care and collecting your medical records.

Jason's comment:

There may be times that you see your dermatologist a lot, so it's important to find one who you can relate to well. Your treatment should be a partnership.

42. What is a "topical" treatment? What is a "systemic" treatment?

Treatments for psoriasis can generally be classified as "topical" or "systemic" based on how the medication reaches psoriatic skin. Topical treatments include creams, lotions, ointments, solutions, or foam directly applied to skin affected by psoriasis. Topical treatments are composed of an **active ingredient** mixed into a vehicle or base, usually a cream or ointment, to allow the active ingredient to enter the skin for treatment. Some forms of light treatment, such as UVB and lasers, have mostly **local effects** and act more like a topical treatment; others, such as PUVA, appear to work both locally and systemically.

Topical treatments are best for small areas of psoriasis, for people who prefer not to take oral medications, and for people who have other illnesses that are being treated at the same time. For most people with psoriasis, topical treatments will control their psoriasis well, and they may never need systemic treatment.

Systemic treatment is given by mouth, by injection, or by intravenous infusion, and reaches the entire body. It is especially useful for patients with moderate or severe psoriasis, or for people with psoriatic arthritis. People with psoriasis scattered all over the body in small spots may prefer systemic treatment because of the length of time needed to treat each small spot with topical treatments. Those with more extensive involvement, associated arthritis, psoriasis that is particularly painful and itchy, or resistant to topical treatment may want to consider systemic treatment. The main disadvantage to this approach is that the entire body is exposed to the medication and therefore affected by the effects and side effects.

43. What are my options for topical treatments?

Fortunately, many different topical treatments are available to treat psoriasis. Your initial choices may

Active ingredient

The ingredient in a topical or oral medicine that is known or expected to have a therapeutic effect.

Local effects

Effects of a medication, either beneficial or unwanted, that appear only at the site of administration. For example, a topical corticosteroid could treat psoriasis locally, or could cause local skin thinning.

depend on recommendations from your doctor, and different therapies are usually used over time.

Topical Steroids

Topical steroids are the mainstay and first choice for mild psoriasis treatment. For most patients, this is the first treatment they will try. Among topical steroids, various types, strengths, brands, and vehicles (the cream, lotion, or ointment that the steroid is mixed into) are available. They are easy and convenient to use and are great for short-term use. Unfortunately, they may lose some effect over time and can cause skin thinning at high doses. It might be helpful to take a break from steroids and use a different treatment for a few weeks in order to improve their effectiveness.

Calcipotriene, Sold as Dovonex and Calcitriol, Sold as Vectical

Calcipotriene and calcitriol are vitamin D analogs approved by the **Food and Drug Administration (FDA)** to treat psoriasis. Calcipotriene is currently available in three formulas—a cream, an ointment, and a solution—all at the same concentration (0.005%). The side effects are generally mild and include stinging skin. It is not recommended for use on the face, near the eyes, or on mucous membranes. For people using calcipotriene on a large body surface area, blood calcium levels may increase. Neither medication has been formally evaluated for use in children. There is also a combination product containing calcipotriene and the steroid betamethasone that is sold as the product **Taclonex** in the United States and as Daivobet in Europe. Its major advantage is that it is approved for once-daily use and may therefore be much easier for some people to use than the component ingredients applied separately up to two times a day.

Food and Drug Administration (FDA)
The federal organization dedicated to protecting the safety of the food and drug supply for the United States.

Taclonex
An ointment made of the combination of calcipotriene and the steroid bethamethsone for use on body psoriasis.

73

Tazarotene, Sold as Tazorac

Tazarotene is a derivative of vitamin A available by prescription as a gel and a cream at two strengths (0.05 and 0.1%) and is approved by the FDA to treat psoriasis, acne, and **photoaging** (aging caused by the sun). It is effective by itself and in combination with topical steroids, light, or calcipotriene. The most common side effect of topical tazarotene is stinging and skin irritation. This irritation may improve with time, but you might need to use the lower strength, use it with a topical steroid, or stop using it for a period of time. Women of childbearing age are strictly advised not to get pregnant while using this medication because it can absorb into the system; a physician may require a pregnancy test before use.

Tar and Its Derivatives

Tar and its derivatives (**crude coal tar**, **anthralin**, and **liquor carbonis detergens [LCD]**) are some of the oldest treatments for psoriasis and continue to be effective and inexpensive. Tar is commonly found in over-the-counter tar shampoos, including Neutrogena T-Gel, some of which are marketed to treat dandruff. There are several commercial tar-based solutions (Psorent), creams, ointments, foams (Scytera), and gels on the market as well, most sold without a prescription. Alternatively, physicians can write a prescription for LCD (in some places a prescription is not required), a form of tar that can be easily mixed at home into a **petrolatum**-based ointment (such as Vaseline) and is a very inexpensive treatment approach.

For psoriasis, anthralin is currently sold over-the-counter in a 1% cream as Psoriatec and in other products for topical use. Because it can be irritating, it is

Photoaging
The naturally occurring aging process that progresses during a lifetime of sun exposure.

Crude coal tar
Under very high temperatures, coal can be destructively distilled to crude coal tar. When applied to skin, coal tar has antibacterial, anti-itching, and photosensitizing properties.

Anthralin
A derivative of tar that is used to treat psoriasis. It decreases skin inflammation but can stain skin and clothing.

Liquor carbonis detergens (LCD)
Crude coal can be refined with alcohol extraction to yield liquor carbonis detergens (LCD). This type of tar therapy works like other tar types to decrease skin inflammation.

often used for short periods and then washed off. Two common regimens are applying it for 10 to 30 minutes before washing off and overnight use of a cream or ointment preparation that is washed off in the morning. Unless the hands are also being treated, they should be washed immediately after touching tar or anthralin. Anthralin should not be applied to skin folds or broken skin. It can stain clothing, towels, bed sheets, and the shower—everything that comes into contact with anthralin needs to be washed immediately, including shower tiles, to prevent brown staining.

Petrolatum

A semisolid mixture of hydrocarbons that is inert and free of water molecules. Vaseline and Aquaphor are commonly used brands of petrolatum. It can be used alone as an ointment or mixed in with other medications.

Treatment

44. Many treatments come in lotion, cream, or ointment form. How do I choose among these?

When comparing many different formations of a specific medication, the ointment formulation is often the most potent. The oil-based ointment formulation creates a barrier over the skin, allowing more medication to penetrate, and is somewhat more resistant to washing and rubbing off.

More sophisticated formulation techniques are changing this pattern, however. For example, foam appears to deliver more active medication than other formulas containing a particular ingredient. This trend is important because most people have very specific preferences about what works best and what feels most comfortable in different areas. It is helpful to try different kinds to find the one that works best for you.

Unfortunately, these preferences mean that a patient will often leave the doctor's office with a handful of prescriptions. It is important to make sure you understand when and where a certain medication should be used on the body. Generally, no more that one topical

It is important to make sure you understand when and where a certain medication should be used on the body.

steroid is usually used on one area of skin. For example, if using a steroid foam on the scalp, there is no reason to use steroid ointment on the scalp as well.

For skin on the body, ointments, creams, and lotions are used most often. If dry skin, cracking, or scaling is a problem, thicker formulations such as ointments and creams can help with the dryness, while bringing medication to affected skin. For those who prefer a more "dry" topical treatment, gel, solution, and foam formulations may be available. Gels, solutions, foams, and other liquids such as medicated shampoos are designed for scalp use, and can reach scalp skin while minimizing accumulation on the hair.

Tip: Label prescription tubes with a marker when you bring them home from the pharmacy. Often, the instructions are on the box, which gets thrown away long before the medicine is used up.

45. I've been prescribed many different topical steroids. Why are there so many, and how do they work?

Corticosteroid

An umbrella term for different steroid compounds. Sometimes called steroids. These may be topical or oral.

Systemic steroids

Steroids that are given orally, by injection, or by vein and therefore have many different effects on the body.

All topical **corticosteroid** (or steroid) preparations work in a similar way by binding to steroid receptors in skin and immune cells, in order to reduce inflammation and cause other effects. The differences lie in the strength of the steroid (see Table 3), the concentration of the steroid, and in the vehicle or material into which it is mixed. Topical steroids work in the same way as **systemic steroids** such as prednisone but in a limited area on the skin. Over 80 different corticosteroid formulations are available.

When using topical steroids, a few commonsense precautions can save time and money, and minimize side effects.

- Use only one steroid in one body area at a given time. For example, if you use one steroid on the body and one on the face, do not switch them or apply both to both places.
- Treat only skin with psoriasis, and try to avoid treating healthy skin.
- Use only a thin layer to treat the skin; only the medication that contacts the skin is absorbed, and the rest rubs off on clothes and sheets.
- If skin is dry, use a moisturizer over the topical steroid instead of using more steroid medication.
- Keep track of how long you are continuously using a topical steroid and whether it continues to be effective.

Hydrocortisone is the mildest and most commonly used topical steroid. It is available in several different strengths over-the-counter and by prescription. Because it is mild, it can be used for a longer time period without skin changes or other side effects. For this reason, it is often mixed into lotions and creams with other medications to treat various skin diseases. Unfortunately, because it is so mild, it does not always improve the appearance of psoriasis.

Like all medications, topical steroids do have side effects. With long-term use, especially in areas with very thin skin such as the eyelids, all steroids have the potential to thin the skin and cause **atrophy**. The risk of atrophy is related to the strength of the steroid, the length of time it is used, and how thin the skin was initially. Areas that are "occluded" (for example, covered by another area of skin such as the armpits and groin) are also particularly susceptible to atrophy. This skin thinning may come with a change in skin color or the appearance of stretch marks and is permanent.

Atrophy
Thinning of the skin that can be an unwanted side effect of topical steroid use. Atrophy decreases the thickness and strength of the affected skin.

77

Another serious side effect of topical steroid use is systemic absorption, when the active steroid is absorbed through the skin and enters the bloodstream. The risk of this effect is related to the strength of the steroid and the amount of steroid used, with super-potent topical steroids most often causing this problem. For super-potent (Class I) steroids, systemic absorption can be seen in people after only 2 weeks of daily use. When steroids are absorbed into the blood, they can suppress the body's natural steroid production. This effect is reversible and subsides as steroids are stopped. Because of this side effect, super-potent steroids are usually reserved for intermittent limited use or as **combination therapy** with nonsteroid medications.

Because steroid side effects can be permanent, it is important to keep track of the type and quantity being used. One way to measure steroid use is by measuring medication used in grams per treatment. If you notice that you are using a large amount of topical steroids or are relying on super-potent topical steroids to control your psoriasis, it could be time to add another topical treatment to your routine (discussed in Question 46). Physicians generally agree that steroids alone aren't usually the most effective long-term way to treat psoriasis. On the other hand, not using enough medication can also be a problem and can limit the effectiveness of these medicines.

Topical Steroid Potency

Some active ingredients, such as betamethasone and hydrocortisone, have multiple formulations at different **potency** based on their chemical makeup. The second word in an ingredient name helps to identify which chemical form is being used. The concentration needed

Combination therapy

Combining two or more treatments to improve effectiveness and in some cases to minimize side effects.

Potency

A way to describe the strength of a medication. It may be measured by the concentration or amount used, or measured, relative to a standard (hydrocortisone for topical steroids).

to achieve certain potency varies depending on the steroid. For example, 1% hydrocortisone is considerably weaker than 0.1% triamcinalone, and betamethasone dipropionate is stronger than the same concentration of betamethasone valerate.

46. I use topical steroids, and after a while they seem to stop working. Why does this occur?

Chronic use of topical steroids can cause them to become less effective. Patients often comment that a topical steroid works very well at first but loses effectiveness over time. Some physicians think that steroids are affected by **tachyphylaxis**—the skin builds resistance to the steroid over time. Others suggest that some people tend to use less topical medication or apply the medications less frequently the longer they use it. While this resistance can be overcome by using stronger formulations, it is usually more effective to stop steroid use for a period of time or add another medication.

Tachyphylaxis

The phenomenon where a medication becomes less effective over a long period of use.

Many people find success using topical steroids in combination with another topical therapy such as calcipotriene or tazarotene. This may involve using one during the day and one at night, one during the week and the other on the weekend, and so forth.

An alternative option is to "pulse" topical steroids. In this scenario, steroids are used consistently and frequently for a short period of time to maximize their beneficial effects. The patient then switches to another regimen for longer-term maintenance therapy.

Another strategy that can make the steroids easier to spread is to mix in a 1:1 ratio with a moisturizer. It dilutes the steroids somewhat but the moisturizer is also beneficial, so the benefits are generally well maintained.

For all treatments of psoriasis, rotational treatment or rotating between different therapies over time can be helpful (discussed in Question 62). Another therapeutic approach used by some dermatologists is a "**therapy holiday.**" This "holiday" may occur in the summer, for example, if sunlight is beneficial, and all other treatments can be stopped for a period of time.

Therapy holiday

A scheduled time without therapy, planned by a patient and his or her physician.

Medications also stop being effective when they are used less frequently.

Medications also stop being effective when they are used less frequently. Studies show that over time people use less and less medication, or use medication less frequently, than right after starting a new medication. As in many chronic skin diseases, people who have had psoriasis for longer time or people who are sad about their disease may tend to use treatments less frequently.

47. Do topical medicines have side effects?

All topical medications, like systemic medications, have side effects. These effects are usually mild but can be very severe and cause life-threatening harm or permanent skin changes.

Systemic effects

Effects of a medication that reach throughout the body and therefore may affect organs or systems beyond the skin or joints.

Side effects can range from local effects that appear where the medication is applied to **systemic effects** that occur when medication is absorbed through the skin. Local effects include redness, itching, stinging, or burning, and usually stop after the medication is washed off or stopped. Systemic effects may take longer to appear. Systemic absorption is increased for people with broken skin and for children and is often related to the medication amount and frequency of use. Covering treated skin with an occlusive bandage can increase a topical treatment's efficacy but may also increase the chance of unwanted effects. Both local and systemic side effects tend to become more frequent as a person uses a medicine to cover more of the body's surface area.

Topical Steroids

Local application can cause impaired wound healing, worsening of any preexisting skin infection, and permanent skin thinning. Skin discoloration, often lightening or reddening of skin tone, can also occur. Like most topical medicines, topical steroids can cause itching and burning. Although rare, an allergy to the medication or the product it is mixed into can develop.

Systemic absorption can cause suppression of a person's own adrenal glands, causing side effects similar to oral prednisone, such as water retention, weight gain, and bone thinning. These side effects can be a problem if the steroids are used in large quantities over extended periods of time. As a guideline, systemic absorption of topical steroids becomes detectable if 50 g of clobetasol proprionate (in the strongest class of steroids) or 500 g of hydrocortisone (in the weakest class of steroids) is used per week. Steroids are typically prescribed in 15-, 30-, and 60-g tubes, and should be labeled clearly so monitoring the amount used can be done easily. Whether from local application or systemic absorption, rapidly stopping topical steroids without adding another treatment can cause psoriasis to flare in some cases.

Calcipotriene (Dovonex) and Calcitrol (Vectical)

After local application, itching, burning, rash, and increased sun sensitivity can occur. The itching usually resolves with time and may decrease after long-term use. Some people's skin may feel dry after application.

Systemic absorption can occur when used in children or when used by adults over a large body surface area. It does not cause problems for most people but can raise blood calcium levels when used over large surface areas.

Tazarotene (Tazorac)

Local application can cause skin irritation such as itching or stinging. In severe reactions, redness and itching may progress to skin peeling.

Systemic absorption does occur, and tazarotene should be clearly avoided during pregnancy because this class of medications is well known to cause serious birth defects. Your physician may require a negative pregnancy test before starting this therapy, and women should stop using tazarotene before trying to conceive.

Tacrolimus and Pimecrolimus

Following application of these treatments, local skin irritation is the most common side effect. Because these medications are used mainly for inverse psoriasis or areas with thin skin, the risk of skin irritation is increased. Both may cause stinging that lasts for a few days after use.

Systemic absorption is rare among adults and children. Both medications are approved for use in adults and children. In infants treated with tacrolimus, detectable blood levels of this **immunosuppressant** have been reported.

Immunosuppressant

Anything that inhibits or weakens the immune system. Immunosuppressants can be drugs, such as prednisone and cyclosporine, or diseases, such as cancer or HIV.

Taclonex

This product is a combination of a potent topical steroid and calcipotriene. The steroid component minimizes the risk of irritation sometimes seen with calcipotriene, but there is still a small risk of atrophy because of the steroid used. It is not recommended for folds or the face as a result.

Minimizing Side Effects

The risk for side effects is highest when applying any topical medication to a large skin area, using multiple medications, or when applying to broken skin. Because it is impossible to know who will experience side effects, it is important to watch the skin carefully.

On the other hand, to maximize the effectiveness of any medication, it is important to use enough medicine, and to use it frequently enough to see results. If you have questions about whether you are using the right amount, be sure to ask your doctor.

Table 4 can help to estimate how much medication should be used on the skin.

48. What is medication compounding? Is it useful to treat psoriasis?

Compounding is the specialized mixing of one or more medications into a cream, lotion, ointment, alcohol, or other base for topical use. Compounds are usually individually mixed based on a doctor's prescription by a specialized pharmacy for a particular person to use.

Compounding
Mixing two or more different medications into a topical cream or ointment.

Compounded formulas for psoriasis may include medications such as:

• A topical corticosteroid to treat inflammation
• Salicylic acid or urea to break up scale

Table 4   Estimating Amount of Topical Medication to Use

Location	One Application	Two Times Daily for 2 Weeks
Hands or face	2 g	60 g
One arm, back, stomach, or chest	3 g	80 g
Entire body	30 to 60 g	840 g to 1680 g

- Menthol or phenol to calm itch
- Tar or tar derivatives to treat inflammation and reduce thickness of plaques

Two or more of these ingredients may be combined in a base of petrolatum (such as Vaseline or Aquaphor), emollient cream (such as Eucerin or Cetaphil), or others.

The advantages of compounding include the ability to mix multiple medicines, the opportunity to use a patient's preferred lotion or cream base with medication, and the flexibility to customize topical treatment for each person.

The advantages of compounding include the ability to mix multiple medicines, the opportunity to use a patient's preferred lotion or cream base with medication, and the flexibility to customize topical treatment for each person.

The main disadvantages of compounding topical medications are the cost and the limited number of pharmacies who are still willing to mix custom medications. Because of the cost, insurance companies may require a letter from your physician prior to covering this medication.

Some dermatologists routinely compound medications. Most tend to use prescribed ointments, creams, and lotions that are already made because of the convenience and consistency of premade medications. If a patient is considering trying a mixture of medicines, the treating dermatologist may be able to suggest a combination therapy for psoriasis and teach simple compounding that can be done at home.

49. How should I clean my skin if I have psoriasis?

There aren't any special cleansing precautions that need to be taken to clean areas of skin affected by psoriasis, but a few caveats may help improve the skin.

The first is to recognize that any cleanser or soap that dries out the skin may make psoriasis worse. Virtually every soap, and even hot water alone, will dry out the skin to some extent. Therefore, it is particularly important to use moisturizers after bathing to help prevent this problem. Some medicated soaps available over-the-counter contain the antifungal and antibacterial zinc pyrithione, such as ZNP soap, and may be helpful to keep psoriasis under control.

When showering and washing, it is important to be gentle with psoriatic skin. At times some people have the urge to aggressively remove scale, but a gentle approach to this and other cleaning can spare the skin unnecessary injury and lead to faster healing. While it can be satisfying, scrubbing with apricot scrubs, sugar or salt scrubs, or a loofah can injure skin and lead to re-appearance of psoriasis.

If the skin breaks or cracks, the urge to disinfect the cracks with alcohol or alcohol-based antibacterial solutions like Bactine should be avoided. Using an antibiotic ointment or even Vaseline by itself will help protect broken skin and help healing without worsening the dryness or causing pain.

50. How can I gently remove scale from the skin?

Scale on the skin and scalp is particularly challenging because of flaking and occasional bleeding that occurs when it is removed. This scale can also be frustrating when it flakes onto hair, clothes, and belongings. Aggressive treatment of psoriasis reduces scale over time, but specific treatments are particularly good at reducing scaling temporarily.

Keratolytics are compounds that break up scale and are present in several lotions, creams, and ointments. These ingredients include lactic acid or lactate (sold as Am-Lactin, Lac-Hydrin, and other brands), urea (sold as Carmol and other brands), salicylic acid (found in many antidandruff shampoos and acne treatments), and other alpha hydroxy acids like glycolic acid. These compounds gently break up the scale and will allow it to shed more quickly. Because some of these products can sting, using moisturizers with these products can be important. A lotion or ointment component can help keep the skin moisturized and reduce painful cracking and fissuring.

Scalp oils are sold under various brand names to remove scale from the scalp. These oils are designed to moisturize the scalp and gently separate the scale from the scalp by penetrating between scale and healthy scalp. The scale is then combed and washed off of the scalp along with the excess oil. The treatment can take over an hour or overnight, and can be repeated as needed to loosen and remove scale. Wearing a plastic shower cap can keep the oils better in place, improve penetration, and reduce the potential mess on sheets and pillows.

One important caution with scalp psoriasis is to learn to ignore the urge to scratch or pick at scaly areas.

One important caution with scalp psoriasis is to learn to ignore the urge to scratch or pick at scaly areas. While scratching at dry scale can be very satisfying, picking and scratching can cause trauma, broken skin, and bleeding. This minor scalp injury slows healing and can even make psoriasis worse through Koebnerization (discussed in Question 30).

51. How can I treat the itchy skin of psoriasis?

Itchy skin is a common and frustrating symptom in psoriasis. It is caused by several factors, including dry flakes of skin that can stretch and crack, scale on the skin, and warm inflamed areas of psoriasis.

The first line of defense against itching is keeping the skin hydrated. Skin with psoriasis usually needs heavy lotions or ointments to stay moist. Heavier, thicker creams such as Eucerin, Neutrogena Norwegian Formula, Aveeno Skin Relief, Cutemol, Dove Cream Oil Intensive Body Lotion, and many others tend to be more effective than lotions and creams with a higher water or alcohol content. Oatmeal, dimethicone, glycerin, lanolin, and petrolatum are ingredients often found in creams that can help with skin moisturizing. Lotions may be less effective because they contain less oil and therefore allow the water content of the skin to evaporate more quickly. Bath oils can be a great way to seal in hydration and are easy to use (although be careful about the slippery tub!). Some favorites are Aveeno Bath Oil and Neutrogena Sesame Seed Shower Oil.

To minimize scale, some lotions or creams come with keratolytics, ingredients that gently loosen and remove scale. Keratolytics include salicylic acid, urea-based compounds, and alpha hydroxy acids such as lactic acid (Eucerin Plus) or glycolic acid.

To calm itching immediately, several approaches can be effective. Topical treatments that provide immediate relief include menthol-based lotions and creams (such as Sarna Lotion, Aveeno Anti-Itch Cream, and Eucerin Calming Itch Relief Treatment), and lotions with topical anesthetics like lidocaine and benzocaine. Menthol, the active ingredient in other creams like Ben-Gay and Tiger Balm, can be soothing to itchy skin. Pramoxine is another anti-itch medication found in creams such as Pramasone and can be found in combination with heavy lotions for use at night. Cooling lotion in the refrigerator before use can help calm itch temporarily, especially during the summer.

Cool compresses, made by dipping a pillowcase, sheet, or towel into warm water and applying to the skin for 10 to 30 minutes, can help relieve itching. It is important to moisturize immediately after applying the compresses because, although water evaporation from the skin relieves itching, it can also dry the skin. An ice pack placed on skin over a towel can provide temporary relief. However, applying ice or a cold pack directly to skin could cause local frost injury so isn't recommended.

An often overlooked cause of itching for people with and without psoriasis is frequent bathing or long showers with hot water. Although hot water feels soothing, water and soaps remove the skin's protective natural oils and can cause or exacerbate skin dryness and irritation. Ways to reduce this irritation include limiting bathing to once per day; shortening showers to 5 minutes or less; showering with warm rather than hot water; using a nonirritating cleanser designed for dry skin such as Cetaphil, Olay Body Wash, or Dove; and applying moisturizer immediately afterward after patting the skin dry. The urge to shower and scrub off skin scale may be strong, but over time one short shower a day before applying cream can reduce skin tightness, dryness, and cracking.

Because many people are most bothered by itching at night, oral medication to calm itching and help sleep can sometimes help. Options include an antihistamine such as Benadryl (diphenhydramine)—available over-the-counter—or Atarax (hydroxyzine), which is available by prescription. Depending on your particular situation and physician's advice, other medications can be prescribed to help with sleep. If you itch at night while you sleep, cotton pajamas that cover irritated skin can protect from unwanted trauma. Consistent skin protection can prevent itching and skin injury due to scratching.

52. My scalp is particularly difficult to treat. What are my options?

People with scalp psoriasis often find that the worst aspect of scalp disease is scalp scaling. To reduce the scale and treat the underlying activity, several medications and preparations are available to treat scalp skin.

Preparations that can be effective on the scalp are:

- Solution: A mixture of medication in water or water and alcohol, usually applied directly onto the scalp around the base of the hair
- Foam: A mixture of medication in an alcohol- or water-based foam dispensed from a pressurized metal canister (similar to hair mousse)
- Ointment: A medication in a petroleum-based ointment similar to Vaseline or petrolatum; best for scalp areas without hair such as behind the ears
- Alcohol-based mixtures of medication in alcohol and water that are compounded by a pharmacy based on a physician's order
- Steroid injections into scalp psoriasis by a physician

Not all medications are available in all formulas, although various strengths of topical steroids are found in all of the above preparations. Newer medications usually come in fewer formulas. Calcipotriene is available as a solution, ointment, or cream, and tazarotene is available as a gel or cream.

In addition to consistently used medications, certain daily routines can help improve scalp psoriasis. Short showers with warm rather than hot water can decrease scalp dryness. Use of gentle, nonirritating shampoos can also help with dryness, and some people find that regular use of over-the-counter antidandruff shampoos can help with scalp scaling.

In addition to consistently used medications, certain daily routines can help improve scalp psoriasis.

Mild hair loss may occur at areas of scalp psoriasis. Hair may fall out after psoriasis appears but will normally grow back because the hair follicles are not permanently damaged. While scalp disease can be very visible and hard to treat, psoriasis on the scalp almost never causes permanent hair loss. Treating scalp psoriasis aggressively can decrease the risk that a person's hair will shed.

53. Is there a way to treat the nail changes of psoriasis?

Psoriatic nails usually have changes such as whitish "oil spots," yellow discoloration, crumbling at the tips called onycholysis, and easy breakage. The "oil spot" appearance is a common characteristic, and is caused by small areas of psoriasis occurring underneath the nail. All nails can be affected, although it occurs more often in fingernails than in toenails. After spots appear on the nail, these changes can't be removed but must grow out completely.

Because fingernails are very visible, and psoriatic nail changes can look similar to nail fungus, people often want to treat their nails to look "normal." To prevent changes in newly growing nail, several options are available. Unfortunately, the nail bed underneath the nail is a challenging area to reach with topical medicines. Systemic therapies for psoriasis, usually prescribed for people with moderate or severe skin disease or psoriatic arthritis, will treat nail changes at the same time. Topical steroids can work as well, and a steroid called flurandrenolide is available in an occlusive dressing sold as Cordran Tape. This tape can be wrapped around the nail bed of the finger to treat the nail and nail bed overnight. Another way to get steroids into the nail bed (at the growing end of the nail, where new nail is being developed) is to inject steroids directly into the skin by the nail bed. These injections can be painful but are able to rapidly deliver steroids to the nail. The injections need to be repeated, often monthly. Some of the biologic agents appear to help with nail disease considerably but generally are not prescribed for this problem alone because the whole body is exposed to the drug when it is given.

Because nails grow slowly (approximately 0.01 inch (0.03 cm) per month, or 5 to 7 months for an average nail), it takes a long time for diseased nails to be replaced by healthy nail. Nail growth is more rapid in summer, in pregnancy, and during sleep. Because of this slow growth, changes may not be seen immediately, and every treatment will take some time to take effect.

Although nail psoriasis is a cause of many characteristic nail changes, it is always possible to have other common nail problems, such as fungus in the nail or abnormal nail growth from previous physical trauma to the nail bed. Nails should be checked by a physician and treated appropriately.

John's comment:

I have severe psoriasis on my nails. "Nail changes" does not really sufficiently describe the physical disfigurement as well as the fragile state of the nails. I've found biological treatments to significantly improve the nails.

54. I have psoriasis on my hands and feet. How can I treat these areas?

Psoriasis on the hands and feet, or palmar-plantar psoriasis, is a particularly challenging type of psoriasis to treat. These locations are often irritated during daily life and can be hard to treat because topical medications work best when given time to absorb. Additionally, the thick skin of the palms and soles can block absorption of topical medicines. Palmar-plantar psoriasis appears as thickened, scaly skin or as pustules under the skin; some people experience both problems.

Topical therapies used for other parts of the body can be used for the hands and feet. Because of the thick skin in these areas, the treatments may need to be stronger or stay on for a longer period of time. Ointments are usually indicated for hands and feet, instead of creams or lotions, and stronger topical steroids can be used. One way to improve topical treatments of hands and feet is to apply ointment, then cover the area with cotton gloves or socks before going to bed. Thin socks and gloves are adequate, and natural fibers such as cotton will prevent further irritation and contact dermatitis. Keratolytics (discussed in Question 51) can also help break down the thick scale to allow other topical medications to penetrate. Using a medication overnight is usually sufficient to treat these areas.

Paint PUVA

A special type of PUVA where psoralen is "painted" directly onto the skin before exposure to UVA light in the same area.

Topical PUVA, sometimes referred to as "**paint PUVA**," can be quite effective for hands and feet. With topical

PUVA, a light-activating medication called **psoralen** is painted on the hands or feet, and the body part is then exposed to a **UVA** light source such as a small hand or foot light box. The advantage of this approach is that only the affected skin is exposed to the psoralen and the UV light, minimizing the chance of sunburn on healthy skin.

For people with severe palmar-plantar psoriasis, systemic therapies can be an effective treatment option (discussed in Question 60).

55. I think I might have psoriasis in the genital area, but I am too embarrassed to ask my doctor. How can I treat it?

Genital psoriasis typically responds to the same types of medication as psoriasis on other parts of the body. However, there are a few very important caveats. First, mid- to high-potency steroids (Classes I to V as listed in Table 3) should NOT be used in the groin because the risk of side effects, such as skin thinning, is much greater. Second, because skin is thinner in the groin region, using medications with thicker bases such as an ointment can be more effective than a lotion of the same medication. Because genital skin is so sensitive, skin irritation could be a problem, and some medications may need to be used less frequently.

One type of topical medication, the topical immuno-modulators such as tacrolimus and pimecrolimus, are an excellent option for genital psoriasis. While not as effective for "regular" psoriasis, this treatment absorbs easily and works well in more sensitive skin of the groin area. These medications do not appear to cause the skin thinning that can sometimes be seen with topical steroids, so they can be a good choice for this area.

Psoralen

A medicine that, when taken by mouth or put onto the skin, increases the skin's sensitivity to UVA light. In combination with UVA light, it is called PUVA and is used to treat psoriasis and other skin diseases.

UVA

A particular wavelength of light that is used in combination with a medication called psoralen to treat psoriasis.

Treatment

56. What is light therapy, and how is it used to treat psoriasis?

Wavelength

The length of a particular wave of light. These lengths vary in different types of light (ultraviolet vs. visible light or different types of UV light, for example) and help determine how far into the skin these waves will penetrate.

It has long been noted that exposure to sunlight helps calm the symptoms of psoriasis.

Ultraviolet (UV) radiation comes naturally from the sun along with visible light. It has a shorter **wavelength**, so it is not visible to the naked eye. It is also the part of sunlight that causes suntan and sunburn. It has long been noted that exposure to sunlight helps calm the symptoms of psoriasis. Even the ancient Greeks recognized it as a treatment for psoriasis. Specialized lights have been developed to deliver UV radiation in precisely measured doses onto a patient's skin in seconds or minutes per session. UV radiation is helpful by itself, and its usefulness can be increased by the addition of psoralen, a pill that increases sensitivity to a specific type of UV radiation called UVA. This medication improves the efficacy of light treatment, but has several disadvantages including increasing the risk of skin cancer and stomach upset. People taking psoralen must also protect their eyes in-between treatments when they are likely to be light sensitive.

The wavelength of therapeutic light sources varies, and the most commonly used wavelengths are UVA (320 to 400 nanometers) and UVB (280 to 320 nanometers). Lights may be referred to as broadband or narrowband, depending on the specificity of the wavelength; both therapies may be used, depending on what equipment is available in a particular city or region.

UV exposure comes most easily from sunlight. Because strong, bright sunlight is not always easily available to all skin and can't be "used" quickly, medical light treatments are available as a substitute (**Table 5**). Different light sources provide varying levels of light: UVB; UVA 1 psoralen, known as PUVA; or narrow-band

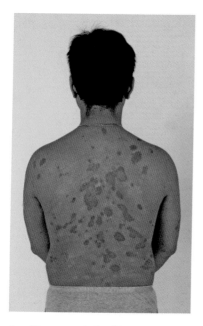

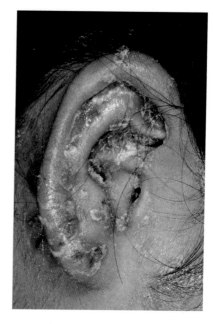

A.   Plaque psoriasis with decreased pigmentation in areas where plaques have resolved.

B.   Scalp and ear psoriasis.

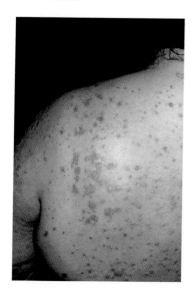

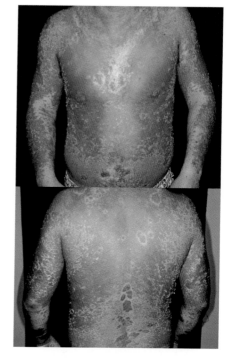

C.   Guttate psoriasis.

D.   Erythrodermic psoriasis.

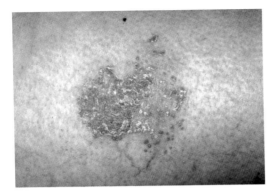

E. Psoriasis caused by use of the medicine interferon.

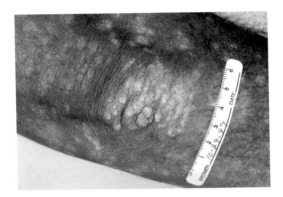

F. Elbow psoriasis with thick scale.

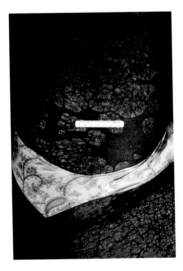

G. Severe plaque psoriasis.

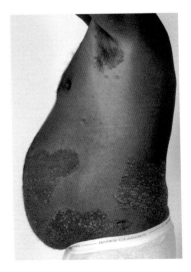

H. Plaque and "inverse" psoriasis with involvement of armpits.

Table 5   Types of UV Therapy

	Availability	Advantages	Disadvantages
Sunlight	Ubiquitous	Very accessible No cost involved	Decreased in winter Skin photodamage over time Dose unknown
UVB	Specialized dermatology offices; home units also available	More widely available than NBUVB Relative safety; risk of UVB may be less than that of the sun	Skin photo damage over time
Narrow-band UVB	Specialized dermatology offices; home units also available	UV radiation is more specific and more effective	Availability of light boxes may be limited in different regions
Psoralen + UVA (PUVA)	Specialized dermatology offices	More effective	Need oral or topical psoralen; skin cancer risk increases with use; no more than 200 treatments recommended over lifetime for people with fair skin; eye protection between visits is important
Tanning bed	Most tanning centers	Generally available	High potential for sun damage to normal skin; mostly UVA light, so not generally as effective as targeted UV
Laser (including Excimer laser)	Specialized dermatology offices	Targeted approach to local psoriasis plaques	Hard to treat large areas; requires repeated visits; costly

UVB (sometimes written NB-UVB). Narrow-band UVA is also under study. All wavelengths of light, given with or without other medications, work by locally decreasing the activity of the immune system cells in the skin, although some may have systemic effects as well.

UVB or PUVA is usually given three to five times a week and takes several months to reach peak effectiveness. Light can be combined with other therapies. When combined with topical therapy, this treatment is often referred to as the **Goeckerman regimen**. When

Goeckerman regimen

A treatment regimen combining topical tar and light therapy, usually performed at designated psoriasis treatment centers.

light is combined with the tar derivative anthralin, it is referred to as the Ingram regimen. Acitretin, a retinoid medicine taken by mouth, is often combined with light, under the name RePUVA. Some reports suggest that alefacept or etancercept may be used effectively in combination with light, and studies combining light with other therapies are also underway.

The long-term risks of UV therapy are similar to those of heavy sunlight exposure. Those who use this therapy may experience skin thinning due to photo damage, also called photoaging, an accelerated version of damage caused by chronic exposure to sunlight. More serious is the increased risk of skin cancers, especially **squamous cell carcinomas** (**SCC**s), which appear to be most common in patients treated with PUVA. The risk of melanoma due to PUVA is low, but this potentially life-threatening skin cancer remains a concern. Non-melanoma skin cancers such as **basal cell carcinomas** (**BCC**s) and SCCs are usually easily treated with timely removal. However, with time, they may spread in one area or, in some extreme cases, metastasize (spread throughout the body) with devastating effects. These risks can be minimized by using strong (SPF of 30 or higher) sunscreen on healthy skin, wearing eye protection, and using thick clothing to cover areas that don't need treatment. For example, thin white cotton boxers may not be adequate to cover the groin area when using a light box. For these reasons, those who use all types of light therapy must be vigilant about checking their skin and about seeing a physician regularly to look for signs of skin cancer. It is important to tell your dermatologist or medical doctor if you have used light therapy in the past, especially PUVA, because increased skin cancer risk is lifelong and remains elevated even after UV treatment.

Squamous cell carcinoma (SCC)

The second most common skin cancer, it arises from the epidermis and resembles the squamous cells that comprise most of the upper layers of skin. This may occur anywhere on the body, including the mucous membranes, but are most common in areas exposed to the sun.

Basal cell carcinoma (BCC)

The most common form of skin cancer. BCC often appears as a small, shiny, raised bump on sun-exposed skin.

Light therapies are most effective for people with large areas of psoriasis, those with scattered smaller spots that are difficult to treat individually, and for disease that resists topical treatment. Care should be taken in people with fair skin who burn easily, with a personal or family history of skin cancer, or who are already exposed to intense sunlight due to work or where they live (where additional sun may not be more effective). Because no central listing of light therapy areas exists, resources such as the National Psoriasis Foundation or your local dermatology society can help you find a local provider.

Light therapies are most effective for people with large areas of psoriasis, those with scattered smaller spots that are difficult to treat individually, and for disease that resists topical treatment.

One way to locate a physician's office or hospital with a light therapy unit is to search the National Psoriasis Foundation's listing of physician providers, which can be searched by type of light therapy and by ZIP code in the United States (see Appendix for more information).

57. What is bath PUVA?

Bath PUVA was developed to take advantage of the benefits of PUVA (oral psoralen 1 UVA) without having to take psoralen internally to activate the UVA light. It is essentially a type of topical PUVA where a person takes a "bath" in a diluted psoralen solution to allow the psoralen to reach the entire body followed by exposure to UVA light. The main advantage is that the risk of eye damage and stomach upset that some people experience after oral psoralen can be almost completely avoided with this approach. The disadvantages are the limited facilities that use this technique and the fact that it is somewhat time-consuming and inconvenient.

Bath PUVA

A type of PUVA therapy where psoralen is washed over the skin in a bath, rather than taken by mouth, before UVA therapy is given.

58. What is psoriasis "day care"?

Psoriasis day care is an all-day outpatient treatment for psoriasis. Initially, psoriasis therapies such as the Goeckerman and Ingram regimens (discussed in Question 56) were developed to be given in the hospital. As medical care moved away from inpatient (overnight) treatment to the outpatient setting, these treatment programs moved out of the hospital. Specialized psoriasis centers were developed to treat patients with tar, anthralin, and light and allowed them to return home at night, leaving their stained clothing at the doctor's office. As co-pays increased, reimbursement by insurance companies decreased, and effective but less time-consuming therapies became available, the number of centers offering "day care" treatment or hospitalization has declined.

There are only a few centers that currently offer this kind of therapy. If the opportunity for an all-day, dedicated treatment location is appealing to you, the National Psoriasis Foundation or other groups can help you to find a center in your area.

59. Can I use sunlight or tanning beds to treat my psoriasis?

If light from the sun or medical UV lamps help your psoriasis, it seems logical that a tanning bed might be helpful as well. For some people, tanning beds supplement the decrease in sunlight over the fall and winter months. However, the primary type of light in a tanning bed is UVA, which is typically not very effective for psoriasis unless combined with light-activating medication. This limitation is one reason why tanning beds don't work as well as receiving light in a doctor's office or from a home UVB light source.

The benefits of tanning beds include wide availability, low cost, and flexible treatment schedules. No physician's appointment, prescription, or co-payment is required, and you can simply stop by your local tanning center for a low-cost visit as needed.

Unfortunately, the convenience and flexibility of this treatment are balanced by its variable effectiveness. Concerns raised about tanning beds include the consistency, intensity, and specificity of the light they supply. Not all units are the same, and each gives a different amount of light depending on the size and number of bulbs it contains. Confounding the problem is the fact that tanning bulbs lose intensity over time, so similarly equipped units (for example, two beds at the same tanning salon) can have different light intensities. Finally, the broad spectrum of light given by these bulbs can increase the amount of non-therapeutic radiation exposure in comparison to specially designed light boxes. Of particular concern are the risks of severe sunburn, which can exacerbate psoriasis through Koebnerization, and the long-term risk of skin cancer, including melanoma.

60. My doctor has recommended systemic treatment for my psoriasis. What are my options, and what are the risks involved?

Systemic treatments are those that reach the whole body though oral or injectable administration (either into a vein, muscle, or the skin). In psoriasis, these treatments are usually used for people with widespread disease, disease that doesn't respond to topical therapy, or skin disease with psoriatic arthritis. All systemic treatments have side effects, but they are important for treating severe disease.

Systemic treatments can be broadly classified into oral therapies such as cyclosporine, methotrexate, and retinoids, and biologic therapies (or "biologics") that are given other ways. The oral therapies for psoriasis are discussed here and summarized in **Table 6**. The biologic therapies are discussed in Question 63.

Methotrexate is one of the oldest therapies for psoriasis and is used commonly to treat a variety of conditions in dermatology and rheumatology.

Liver biopsy

The removal of a small piece of tissue from the liver using a special needle. The tissue is then examined under a microscope to look for the presence of inflammation or liver damage.

Methotrexate is one of the oldest therapies for psoriasis and is used commonly to treat a variety of conditions in dermatology and rheumatology. When methotrexate was first given as a daily medication, it clearly improved psoriasis but was also fairly toxic. Pulse dosing once a week—a technique developed in the 1960s—proved to be an effective and safer alternative, and is still the mainstay of therapy used to treat skin disease today. The main concern with long-term methotrexate use is that high cumulative doses can cause permanent scarring of the liver. People with diabetes seem to be at higher risk for these kinds of complications. For most patients, this means regular laboratory monitoring and possibility of a **liver biopsy** (discussed in Question 61) after taking 1.5 g of the medicine. For most patients, it takes about 3 years of continuous treatment to get to this time point. Another common side effect is stomach upset; taking a folate supplement with methotrexate can help with this problem.

Cyclosporine is a powerful immunosuppressant, often used to treat organ transplant patients to prevent them from rejecting a new heart or kidney. In much lower doses it is exceptionally effective at treating psoriasis. The main side effects that limit its use are high blood pressure and loss of kidney function. Careful monitoring is required, and limiting the duration of use is usually recommended.

Acitretin is a vitamin A derivative that is approved for the treatment of severe psoriasis. It is believed to treat psoriasis by targeting retinoid receptors in the skin that control the growth cycle of skin cells. Acitretin can normalize skin cell growth. Since it does not interfere with the body's immune system, acitretin can be a

Table 6 Systemic Medications for Psoriasis

Medication	How Taken	Monitoring	Pregnancy Category*	Advantages	Cautions
Methotrexate	Several pills once per week; alternatively can be given as intramuscular injection	Liver function tests and blood counts monthly to every several months	X	No direct effects on the kidney; inexpensive, decades of experience with this medication	May require a liver biopsy after several years of use; alcohol intake not recommended during use; risk of bone marrow suppression and infection
Cyclosporine (sold as Neoral and Sandimmune) www.novartis.com	Pill twice per day	Kidney function, urine, blood count, liver tests: checked biweekly, later monthly. Blood pressure and sometimes cholesterol/triglycerides also monitored	C	Generally rapidly effective; no direct effects on the liver	Risk of kidney damage and immunosuppression balanced against benefit for long-term use; may cause increased hair growth on body or increased growth of gums; use not recommended for longer than 1 year
Acitretin (sold as Soriatane) www.soriatane.com	One pill each day, taken with food	Liver function, blood count, fasting cholesterol/lipids: weekly if levels are unstable, later monthly; two pretreatment pregnancy tests, then pregnancy test monthly if pregnancy is possible	X	Does not suppress immune system; effective for pustular and palmar-plantar psoriasis; side effects generally reversible	High cholesterol and lipids in some people, bone changes; dry skin, eyes, and lips, thin hair and nails; liver inflammation; pregnancy not recommended for at least 3 years after use because of known fetal abnormalities; must use two forms of contraception; limit alcohol consumption while using

*Pregnancy categories are established by the FDA. A drug listed as category X is one in which studies have shown that the risk of harm to the fetus clearly outweighs potential benefits. Category C drugs are those in which animal studies show a potential adverse effect for the fetus, but benefits may outweigh risks. See Table 8, p. 132.

good choice for people who are at increased risk of infection. It can also be used successfully in combination with other therapies, especially phototherapy. Acitretin does cause side effects such as inflammation of the liver and elevated triglyceride levels (levels of fat in the blood), so patients should have regular blood tests. It is almost never used in women of childbearing age because this class of drugs is well known to cause serious birth defects and may remain in the body for up to 3 years.

Other systemic medications that have been used for psoriasis with reported success in some people include hydroxyurea, sulfasalazine, mycophenolate mofetil (CellCept), and tacrolimus.

61. What is a liver biopsy?

A liver biopsy is a procedure that may be used to evaluate a person's liver after taking methotrexate over long periods. The American Academy of Dermatology recommends that patients who have received 1.5 g of methotrexate (usually over 2 to 3 years of treatment) undergo this test to make sure that their liver has not been permanently damaged. Some dermatologists may recommend a liver biopsy at this point; others may recommend an evaluation by a **gastroenterologist** (digestive system and liver specialist), and still others may defer this test if all other liver tests are normal.

Gastroenterologist

A physician who specializes in diseases of the digestive tract, gall bladder, and liver.

During a liver biopsy, a gastroenterologist will remove a small sample of the liver with a long needle for examination under the microscope. It is typically an outpatient procedure performed under local anesthesia, and most people go home the same day. A major potential complication from this procedure is bleeding;

the liver is supplied by many blood vessels and bleeds easily. If the results of the biopsy are normal, this can indicate that a person has tolerated methotrexate without permanent complications. If the biopsy shows liver damage, however, changing therapy is usually recommended.

62. What are rotational, combination, and sequential therapies?

Rotational therapy describes the idea that rotating between different psoriasis therapies can maximize their effectiveness while minimizing treatment side effects. Many people rotate therapies over time; however, some work with their physician to plan rotations between therapies on a set schedule.

Rotational therapy
Rotating different therapies over time in order to maximize benefits while minimizing side effects that might accumulate.

Although it's not predictable whether psoriasis will become resistant to a specific treatment over time, rotating therapies can address this possibility with planned therapy switches. A common rotation of therapies is to use UV therapy in the winter and rotate to another treatment in the summer when natural sunlight is more abundant.

The benefits of rotational therapy are greatest when rotating between therapies with different non-overlapping side effects. For example, if a person uses cyclosporine for a period of time, kidney injury is a concern, but with UVB therapy, the major side effect is chronic sun damage. Although neither may be ideal, rotating the exposure to different risks can help minimize the chance of developing a significant problem. A person rotating between UVB and PUVA, for example, of which both cause chronic sun damage, would not necessarily see the same benefit.

Combination therapy describes the scheduled use of two or more medications at the same time or on the same schedule to maximize their benefits while limiting side effects. Sometimes the use of two medications, such as acitretin and light, has shown more benefit than would be expected from either alone, an effect sometimes described as **synergism**.

Synergism
When the benefits of two medications used together are even greater than what they would be if they were simply added because they complement each other in some way.

One popular combination therapy is to use a vitamin A or D analog (tazarotene, calcipotriene, or calcitriol) twice daily on weekdays and a super-potent topical steroid "pulse" on weekends. In this case, the use of a nonsteroid therapy augments the efficacy of the steroid, while minimizing the risk of using a strong steroid for an extended period of time. An additional benefit combining topical steroids with vitamin A or D derivatives is that they minimize any irritation as well as treat psoriasis.

Although the approach is generally quite effective, not all medications can be used in combination. As was previously mentioned, combining steroids to treat the same area of skin at one time is not likely to be helpful. For other combinations, one medication can block the effectiveness of the other. For example, if you are using salicylic acid to treat scaly skin, the acid will break down calcipotriene, eliminating its effectiveness. Formulas containing lactic acid and hydrocortisone valerate also inactivate calcipotriene. Likewise, topical tar will inactivate topical anthralin.

Sequential therapy
Transitioning from one therapy to another to maximize certain treatment characteristics. An example would be starting with a medication that works rapidly to initiate clearing and following it with a slower-acting medication that may be safer for long-term use.

Sequential therapy schedules medicine use and medicine changes to first clear psoriasis and then transition over to a maintenance routine. The sequences are divided into a clearing phase, a transitional phase, and a maintenance phase. Intuitively, this approach is logical for quickly clearing psoriasis and then maintaining therapy over time.

Therapy used during the clearing phase is usually fast acting but may be desirable to use only for a short time. During the transitional phase, a second therapy is introduced while the first is maintained. Finally, the fast-acting therapy is weaned, and the second therapy is continued for long-term maintenance.

In one example, cyclosporine could be used to rapidly clear psoriasis. Acitretin, a drug with different side effects, is then introduced. Acitretin has a slower onset but can often be used for longer periods of time. Cyclosporine is then gradually discontinued, and acitretin will be used alone for maintenance. Light therapy can then be added periodically if additional treatment is needed.

63. I've read about biologic therapies for psoriasis. How do these work?

Sue's comment:

The topical medications were difficult for me. The amount of surface area I had to carefully coat with a thin amount of greasy whatever was impossible. I usually had three types of medications: one for the general surface area, one for the scalp, and a different one for the "skin folds." It was awful. I was discouraged. Not all of the pharmacies carry the psoriasis medications. I had to go to different pharmacies for different medications. I could try to pace the use of my meds to conform to 30-day supplies, but sometimes I would run out. Then I would have to go without meds until I could get a refill. Then there were the side effects of the meds—and there are lots, not to mention the total discomfort from some of the greasy and oily products and the messes to clean up on clothes, bedding, furniture, everywhere.

I tried oral meds. Not much help from one, but lots of help from a different med. Unfortunately, the prescribing info limited me to a year of this med. And I also had to have weekly blood tests to track whether there were any adverse impacts to my liver.

How does it feel now that I am taking a biologic? It is bizarre. I have a hard time remembering that I have psoriasis. I have almost completely clear skin. I don't have flakes all over the car anymore. My sheets stay clean. My showers are entirely comfortable. I can wear short sleeves in 100 degree weather. I can do normal things again.

Biologic therapies, or biologics for short, are proteins that modify the immune system response. These types of medicine were developed to specifically target the immune cells that cause psoriasis by either suppressing the activated immune cells or by stopping the immune cell, signals from causing psoriasis. All of these proteins are designed to interact very specifically with proteins or chemicals found naturally in the blood.

All of these medications have been developed in the past decade or so. Therefore, the full potential and the full risks of these drugs are not yet known. However, the good news is that the effectiveness of these medications appears to be as good as, and in some cases better than, traditional systemic therapies, with fewer side effects and considerably lower risk of damaging other organs such as the liver or kidneys over time. People also feel better in general while they are on them as they don't tend to cause nausea or headaches that are sometimes seen with methotrexate and cyclosporine, for example.

Although these medications work in different ways, they have several things in common. Thus far, all are administered directly into the body by injection or by intravenous infusion, rather than by mouth. Like all therapies that affect the immune system, biologics cause some degree of immunosuppression, which brings with it an inherent risk of new infections.

The optimal way to use these drugs has not yet been established in some cases, so physicians often use personal experience to design a treatment plan for a given individual. The principles of consistent, correct therapy use, proper follow-up, careful observation, and close contact with a physician are important factors when using biologics or any drugs. When using new medications, these principles are essential to minimize potential side effects and maximize the beneficial effects of treatment.

The costs of these medications and required laboratory monitoring can range from $16,000 to $25,000 per year. The cost of some or all of the medication, as well as the cost for monitoring side effects, is usually covered by insurance. For this and other reasons, some insurance companies might require trying other systemic medications or light therapy before introducing these medicines.

More information will be available in the future, but it is clear that these medications represent a huge advance in the search for targeted, specific therapy for psoriasis and other autoimmune diseases.

Like all therapies that affect the immune system, biologics cause some degree of immunosuppression, which brings with it an inherent risk of new infections.

64. What are alefacept and efalizumab?

Alefacept was the first of two biologic therapies to be approved for treating psoriasis in 2003. This medication works by selectively eliminating pathogenic T cells in the body. Alefacept is injected into a muscle once a week, for a total of 12 weeks. Most patients feel well while using it, but all people must be monitored with blood draws for a drop in T cell levels. Alefacept is fairly slow acting, so many physicians are trying it in combination with other therapies to speed up the improvements that patients experience. Although this medicine doesn't work for everyone, people who respond well may be able to go for months without needing any additional therapy.

Efalizumab

A biologic therapy used to treat moderate to severe psoriasis by inhibiting T cells. Previously sold under the trade name Raptiva.

Efalizumab was the second biologic agent approved in 2003. It inhibits inflammatory cell function in the body and is administered through a subcutaneous injection once a week on a continuous basis. Because of reports of a few patients who were affected with a rare infection called progressive multifocal leukoencephalopathy, it was withdrawn from U.S. and European markets in 2009.

65. What are infliximab, etanercept, adalimumab, and golimumab?

These four medications are in a class of drugs described as TNF-α inhibitors. Tumor necrosis factor alpha, or TNF-α, is an important player in the immune system, and decreasing its activity has substantial beneficial effects on both psoriasis and psoriatic arthritis. Suppressing the immune system by any means, however, can increase the risk of serious infection. Although the additional risk associated with these drugs is not large, if you are taking one and don't feel well, you should alert your physician. There may also be some increased risk for some types of skin cancers with these drugs so have your dermatologist keep an eye on any changing spots. One of the main advantages of this class of drugs is that it has been around for more than a decade. As a result there is a large amount of safety information about the class and how to use them. Some physicians have found that when people don't do well on one, they may still improve on another so may try them in series.

Etanercept is approved to treat psoriasis and psoriatic arthritis. Etanercept is injected under the skin once or twice a week with a syringe "pen." The recommended regimen is to start at a higher dose for 3 months (two injections per week), tapering to half the dose for continued treatment. Some people may find, however, that they need to be maintained at a higher dose to remain clear, while others can be maintained on lower doses over time. Studies have been done showing that the medication is straightforward to stop and restart if needed, and the response to the medication is very predictable. No blood tests are required while on this treatment, but physicians will screen for tuberculosis before starting this drug and may also test for other conditions throughout treatment. This is the only one of the systemic drugs to have been studied rigorously in children with psoriasis, in whom it works very similarly to how it works in adults. Etanercept is currently approved for use in children as young as 2 years for other indications.

Infliximab is approved to treat psoriasis and psoriatic arthritis. It was originally developed to treat Crohn's disease. Patients with psoriasis are approximately seven times more likely than those who do not have psoriasis to develop Crohn's disease. This occurrence helped lead to the observation that patients with psoriasis respond dramatically and quickly to this therapy. Infliximab is usually started with an infusion directly into the bloodstream, followed by another infusion 2 weeks later, another infusion 4 weeks later, and then every 2 months.

Patients with psoriasis are approximately seven times more likely than those who do not have psoriasis to develop Crohn's disease.

This regimen may vary, and each infusion lasts approximately 2 to 3 hours. A test for prior exposure to tuberculosis is required prior to starting this medication. Mild reactions during the infusion can occur, but serious reactions are very rare. There have been some reports of liver inflammation on this medication so some doctors also routinely check tests for this. Of the drugs in this class, infliximab is usually the fastest to clear people.

Adalimumab is a third member of this class approved for psoriasis and psoriatic arthritis. Adalimumab is injected under the skin weekly or every other week. It is somewhat more effective in clearing skin psoriasis than etanercept but not quite as good as infliximab in early phases of treatment. All three drugs perform similarly in treating psoriatic arthritis. A test for prior exposure to tuberculosis is required before starting this medication, but no routine laboratory studies are recommended.

Golimumab is the newest of the approved TNF agents in the U.S. market. At the time of publication, golimumab was approved for psoriatic arthritis. This drug has the advantage of being given only once a month and appears to also work in skin psoriasis although it hasn't been tested in a dedicated skin psoriasis study. Because it acts through the same pathway as the other TNF-α inhibitors, both the risks and benefits of this medication are likely to be similar to others in the class.

Information on the biologics and other treatments for psoriasis is changing rapidly as new data from studies are updated and published. **Table 7** summarizes some of the basic differences between the medications, but for the most up-to-date information, please talk with your physician. All of these drugs have Web sites with additional safety information as well.

Table 7   Biologics for the Treatment of Psoriasis and Psoriatic Arthritis

	Adalimumab	Alefacept	Etanercept	Infliximab	Simponi	Stelara
Brand name (manufacturer)	Humira (Abbott)	Amevive (Biogen)	Enbrel (Amgen)	Remicade (Centocor)	Golimumab (Centocor)	Ustekinumab (Centocor)
Web site	*www.humira.com*	*www.amevive.com*	*www.enbrel.com*	*www.remicade.com*	*www.simponi.com*	*www.stelarainfo.com*
How it works	Inhibits TNF-α	Reduces activated T cells	Inhibits TNF-α	Inhibits TNF-α	Inhibits TNF-α	Inhibits Interleukin 12 and 23
FDA-approved uses as of publication date	Rheumatoid arthritis, psoriatic arthritis, psoriasis, ankylosing spondylitis, Crohn's disease, juvenile idiopathic arthritis	Psoriasis	Psoriasis, psoriatic arthritis, rheumatoid arthritis, juvenile idiopathic arthritis (down to 2 years of age), ankylosing spondylitis	Rheumatoid arthritis, psoriatic arthritis, psoriasis, ulcerative colitis, ankylosing spondylitis, adult and pediatric Crohn's disease	Psoriatic arthritis, ankylosing spondylitis, rheumatoid arthritis	Psoriasis
Route of administration and typical schedule	Self-injection every other week or every week	Injection weekly for 12-week cycle in doctor's office	Self-injection 1 to 2 times per week	Infusion into vein every 2 to 8 weeks	Self-injection every month	Injection every 12 weeks
Monitoring (based on FDA recommendations; physician practice may vary)	PPD prior to starting therapy	Blood counts every other week during 12-week treatment cycle	PPD prior to starting therapy	PPD prior to starting therapy Liver function tests	PPD prior to starting therapy	PPD prior to starting therapy

(continued)

Treatment

111

Table 7   Biologics for the Treatment of Psoriasis and Psoriatic Arthritis (Continued)

	Adalimumab	Alefacept	Etanercept	Infliximab	Simponi	Stelara
Pregnancy Category	B	B	B	B	B	B
Advantages	Rapid improvement of psoriasis and effective for psoriatic arthritis	Some people achieve long-lived remissions	Large safety data base; predictable response; straightforward to stop and restart treatment if needed	Large safety data base; rapid onset; large percentage of patients respond well	Approved for psoriatic arthritis, also appears to help psoriasis. General actions of this class well known; infrequent injections	Rapid improvement of psoriasis and effective for psoriatic arthritis New class—may be helpful for people who are resistant to TNF-α alpha inhibitors. Infrequent dosing may be convenient for some people.
						Newest drug, limited safety information
Cautions: All should be used with caution in people who are immunosuppressed or prone to chronic or recurrent infections	Not recommended for people with congestive heart failure; preexisting or newly diagnosed multiple sclerosis; must be tested for tuberculosis prior to starting	Relatively slow onset; only some people respond well Approximately 10% of people will need to stop this medication at least temporarily because of low CD4 T-cell counts	Not recommended for people with congestive heart failure; preexisting or newly diagnosed multiple sclerosis; must be tested for tuberculosis prior to starting	Not recommended for people with congestive heart failure; preexisting or newly diagnosed multiple sclerosis; must be tested for tuberculosis prior to starting	New drug; relatively small amount of safety data available; not recommended for people with congestive heart failure; must be tested for tuberculosis prior to starting	

66. What are ustekinumab (Stelara) and briakinumab?

These two drugs are in a new class of drugs known as IL12-23 or "p40" inhibitors. Interestingly, they were originally developed to suppress the chemical inter-leukin 12, which is key in the immune system. Later, as scientists discovered that there was another key cytokine (interleukin 23) in these diseases, they also found that there was a common part to both chemicals called p40. Fortunately, these drugs target p40 so affect both chemicals. Like all the biologics, they work by affecting the immune system and carry with them a theoretical risk of increased infection. Because this class of drugs is newer, there is less known safety information about them.

Ustekinumab is now approved in the U.S., Canada, and Europe and dosed as an injection under the skin every 12 weeks after an initial loading dose 1 month apart. Heavier patients may qualify for a higher dose. Similar to other biologics, patients don't have many immediate side effects while on the treatment and most have a good response. Further safety data are being collected.

Briakinumab, previously known as ABT-874, is currently in late-phase studies and also appears to be quite effective with an intermittent dosing regimen and similar safety profile.

67. What other new medications are being studied?

Many new medications are being developed to treat psoriasis and are currently in **clinical trials**. Some are new immunosuppressives and others are variations of current medications, such as the vitamin A and vitamin

Clinical trial
A formally designed, officially reviewed scientific study of diagnosis, treatment, intervention, or prevention of a particular disease.

113

D derivatives. Fortunately, there is tremendous current interest in developing novel approaches, and new options are likely to continue to emerge. The National Psoriasis Foundation, American Academy of Dermatology, and the popular press are good places for up-to-date information released at dermatology meetings and in new publications.

68. What does it mean when a medication is FDA approved?

FDA approval is usually a 5- to 7-year process during which a drug maker tests a new therapy in people. Every prescribed and over-the-counter medication, with the exception of supplements and vitamins, requires approval by the FDA before it can be sold in the United States. Most medications are tested in several thousand people before approval. When being considered for approval, a drug's side effects are evaluated against its effectiveness, the severity of the disease being treated, and other options already on the market.

Drugs are evaluated by the FDA based on the results of clinical trials.

Drugs are evaluated by the FDA based on the results of clinical trials. These trials test a medication in a particular group of people (those with moderate to severe psoriasis, for example), and the FDA may grant approval based on these results. During this process, medications are approved for a specific **indication** or disease.

Indication

A symptom, like itching, or condition, like psoriasis, that can be treated through the use of a specific medical treatment or procedure.

69. Can my doctor prescribe something that isn't FDA approved? Is that safe?

Once a drug is approved by the FDA, physicians have the discretion to prescribe it for any indication they decide is necessary. For example, golimumab, a drug approved for psoriatic arthritis, might be prescribed for someone with skin psoriasis only. This practice, called **off-label prescribing**, is allowed under law. Because most drugs are only approved for a few indications, it is common and accepted practice to use medications "off label" in dermatology. In many cases, there are studies to support this use, even if the drug isn't officially approved to be used in this way. The safety of using a drug on a group of people that is different than the group the drug was tested on will depend on characteristics of the two diseases and the underlying health of the two groups. Most of the time, insurance companies and Medicare cover prescriptions for off-label use, although the insurance company or Medicare may ask for information supporting its use. Exceptions may occur when medications are very costly or have severe side effects.

Off-label prescribing

The common and accepted practice of using a prescription medication for a purpose other than the one for which it was approved.

Treatment

Drugs that are not approved by the FDA are not available for sale in the United States. Such drugs are not carried in pharmacies and cannot be prescribed by a physician. These drugs include experimental therapies, which may be available only through research studies, and medications that are available by prescription or for sale in a foreign country or on a foreign Web site. Drugs and products not approved for use in the United States can be offered for sale on the Internet. To see whether a drug is approved by the FDA, search the FDA's online drug list at www.fda.gov.

70. What is a clinical trial?

In general, a clinical trial is a formally designed program to study the effects of a particular drug or intervention (such as light therapy or behavioral changes) on psoriasis or other diseases. Clinical trials come in many formats, and may study prevention, treatment, or a cure for different diseases.

When a new drug is being developed or an old drug is being studied to treat a different disease, a clinical trial is the best way to determine whether a therapy is effective. These trials are required by the FDA prior to new therapy approval but also may be done to test a drug used for an off-label purpose (discussed in Question 69).

In psoriasis, clinical trials can investigate new topical, systemic, or biologic therapies (discussed in Questions 43, 60, and 63). Other trials may investigate already approved therapies in new combinations or therapies currently approved for other uses. After FDA approval, drugs can continue to go through clinical trials to show that they are effective in other diseases.

Although there is no one central resource for all clinical trials, several sources are very comprehensive. The FDA maintains a listing of clinical trials at www.clinicaltrials.gov (see Appendix for more information). The National Psoriasis Foundation lists promising new trials under the "Research" section of their site. A useful feature of both sites is the ability to find clinical trials in a particular city or part of the country. Other searchable databases are listed in the Appendix.

Why do people participate in clinical trials? The answers are varied but usually stem from hope for future therapies. Many people participate in the hope that new information will help others with psoriasis in the future. Some are interested in early access to potential new therapies. Although there is no guarantee of benefit for participating in a clinical trial, the knowledge gained can help others with psoriasis.

There is typically no fee for an individual to participate in a clinical trial. However, some clinical trials will reimburse or pay patients for their time and participation. The payment ranges from reimbursement for travel, parking, and time, to large payments ($1000 or more) for complex studies involving multiple tests, clinic visits, and investigational medications. Because each study is different, it is important to clarify these facts on a study-by-study basis.

Most clinical trials are conducted by university medical centers, doctors' offices, or pharmaceutical companies. The safety and ethics of studies in the United States are critically reviewed by an independent **Institutional Review Board**, or IRB. An IRB is a federally mandated committee made up of doctors, nurses, and community members who review the safety, ethics, and **informed consent** process (the process by which a person learns about a study and agrees to participate).

When learning about a clinical trial, be sure to find out as much information as possible. Make sure you understand which therapies are standard and which are experimental. Confirm that you are able to participate in the study before joining. You will most likely receive a lengthy informed consent agreement to sign. If it is difficult to read or understand, take it home to review before signing it. During your time in a clinical trial, you will see a research doctor and join a research group for your psoriasis. When the trial ends, you can resume care from your usual doctor.

71. Who is eligible for treatment in a clinical trial?

Every clinical trial will have **eligibility criteria**—things that are required or not allowed when participating in a study. These criteria include qualifications for and exclusions to participating in a clinical trial and vary

Treatment

Institutional Review Board (IRB)

Institutional Review Boards, or IRBs, review research studies that involve human participants. They ensure the ethical and safe treatment of study participants.

Informed consent

A document that outlines a person's participation in a clinical trial. Each participant in a clinical trial in the United States must sign a consent form that explains the purpose of the trial, the results expected, how the trial works, potential risks, and a list of other treatments that are available.

Eligibility criteria

In a clinical trial, the criteria that a patient needs to meet in order to participate. Examples include being over age 18 or not planning to become pregnant during the study.

depending on the type of treatment being studied. For example, most biologic and systemic therapy studies seek patients with moderate or severe psoriasis, defined by body surface area or **PASI score** (discussed in Question 72). Common exclusion criteria (factors that prevent an individual from joining a study) include being younger than 18, having other significant illnesses or previous history of cancer, or planning a pregnancy.

PASI Score

A specialized way to measure changes in psoriasis severity used in research studies. It incorporates psoriasis area and psoriasis activity (redness, thickness, and scale). PASI 75 indicates a 75% improvement in the PASI score, often used to track improvement in studies of new medications; PASI 50 is a 50% improvement in the PASI score.

72. My doctor discussed body surface area and PASI scores in psoriasis. What are these?

While it is not hard to tell when psoriasis gets better or worse, researchers testing new therapies have developed ways to measure these changes systematically over time. Many of the recent studies reporting on the effectiveness of a medication use specific measurements of psoriasis, and these measurements can also be important in determining eligibility to participate in a study.

The most straightforward way to measure psoriasis is to measure how much of the body surface area, or BSA, is affected by psoriasis.

In order to describe how severe psoriasis is, a doctor may measure skin disease in several different ways. The most straightforward way to measure psoriasis is to measure how much of the body surface area, or BSA, is affected by psoriasis. Another way is to use the Psoriasis Area Severity Index, or PASI, which combines BSA with a rating of how severe the scaling, thickness, and redness are in a particular area. Two variants of the PASI often used to report research results are the percentage of people at PASI-75 or at PASI-50. A person reaches a PASI-75 or PASI-50 when his or her skin's PASI score has decreased by 75% or 50%, respectively, compared to pretreatment levels. It is significant to note that a PASI-75 represents more than a 75% overall improvement to patients, and most people who reach this level are clear or almost clear of their disease.

The PASI and its variants are preferred to BSA measurements because researchers recognize that the goal for therapy is not just reduction in the size of psoriatic areas but reduction of redness, thickness, and scale in remaining areas as well.

A few quick estimating tools are useful to determine body surface area:

1. Palm rule: The "palm rule" uses the fact that a person's palm (excluding fingers) is about as large as 1% of his body surface area. By adding the number of palm areas affected by psoriasis all over the body, you can find an estimate of the BSA affected by psoriasis.

2. The "Rule of 9s": The Rule of 9s estimates body surface area affected by dividing the body into 11 equally sized skin areas that each comprise about 9% of the body: the head, chest, abdomen, back, buttocks, and on each side, the arm, front of leg, and back of leg.

   A patient or physician can estimate the amount of body surface area affected by adding up the number of regions affected or the amount affected in each area (one-half of the head would be about 5% of BSA).

3. PASI score: The PASI score takes the body surface area and multiplies the BSA by a severity measurement, reflecting how badly affected the area is. In this way, a mildly red-colored spot can be distinguished from a thick, scaly spot by a different score.

The three physical characteristics that are measured include redness (also called **erythema**), thickness (also referred to as **induration**), and scaliness or scale. These characteristics are each rated from 0 (no change) to 4 (most severe) for each body area. Areas such as the

Erythema

A medical term referring to redness of the skin due to blood vessel dilation.

Induration

A medical term for thickening of the skin, as sometimes seen in psoriasis.

119

scalp tend to be more scaly, and elbows and knees tend to be more red and thickened.

Although these measurements aren't used routinely and aren't necessary for patients with psoriasis, they are useful for describing the exact severity of psoriasis and determining eligibility to participate in some clinical trials. Studies have shown that patients are very good at tracking their own progress with a similar set of measurements, which may be a good way to tell whether a treatment is working well.

To be eligible for studies using systemic agents, participants often need about 10% of their body surface area affected and/or a PASI score of 10. This is also a reasonable guide that can be used, for example, to help someone using topical treatments to determine whether more aggressive treatment might be appropriate for them.

73. Which complementary or alternative therapies are available for psoriasis?

Complementary therapy

An umbrella term, sometimes used interchangeably with "alternative therapy," that describes nonprescription medicines, supplements, and disease therapies.

Many **complementary therapies** or alternative therapies are marketed to help treat psoriasis. These therapies are intended to treat the skin directly, to affect the immune system, or to reduce a person's stress level. Some have been formally studied in people with psoriasis, while others are recommended based on the experience of a few individuals.

Some approaches that have been proven to help psoriasis:

- Stress reduction approach, known as mindfulness meditation-based stress reduction therapy
- Psychotherapy
- Stress management, including guided imagery and relaxation

Herbal supplements that have been studied to treat psoriasis:

- Curcumin: A component of the spice tumeric found in curry powder. Curcumin has been studied to treat diseases of the skin including psoriasis both in oral and topical forms. It appears to work as an anti-inflammatory to calm redness and swelling in the skin. The most comprehensive study evaluated oral curcumin in a group of nine patients; of these, two patients saw complete improvement and no person had adverse reactions.
- Indigo naturalis: A dark-blue powder from the leaf of the indigo plant. Indigo naturalis has also been evaluated to treat psoriasis. Several studies of its topical use have been performed, the most recent using an ointment base to apply indigo topically. A recent study in 42 psoriasis patients showed it to be much more effective than ointment alone when comparing medicated ointment to plain ointment on R and L sides for a 3-month period. Of course, the ointment is a blue color and can stain skin or clothing.
- Other supplements that have been studied include Tuhuai extract, licorice extract, Radix Rubiae from the India madder root, and many others. Over time more evidence will likely become available.

Approaches that have been recommended, with limited data:

- Acupuncture
- Traditional Chinese medicine: A broad term that includes an Asian system of healing that seeks to achieve internal balance. Practitioners use methods such as acupuncture, heat application (moxibustion),

herbal preparations, and exercises (tai chi, qigong) to restore the flow of qi (vital energy) and the balance of yin and yang.

- Meditation, including mindfulness-based stress reductions, as well as other types, has been shown to be helpful.
- Massage is helpful for people with psoriasis, psoriatic arthritis, or high levels of stress from any cause, and all can benefit from therapeutic massage.
- Yoga can reduce stress for people with psoriasis and may be beneficial to improve flexibility for those with psoriatic arthritis.
- Climactic therapy: Traveling to a warmer and sunnier climate for 2 to 4 weeks has shown effectiveness for people living in cold environments such as Scandinavia.
- Hypnosis for psoriasis appeared to be beneficial in a group of 11 people studied at Johns Hopkins School of Medicine.

The word "natural" is appealing, but does not guarantee that a therapy is free from risks or side effects.

74. Are there risks to complementary and alternative therapies?

Although alternative or complementary therapies offer hope for psoriasis treatment, like all therapies they include risks and benefits that should be considered. The word "natural" is appealing, but does not guarantee that a therapy is free from risks or side effects.

Major issues in evaluating **alternative therapy** include:

- Effectiveness: Does it work? How has it been tested?
- Safety: Does it have side effects or drug interactions with other medications?

Alternative therapy

Also called complementary therapy. An umbrella term for nonprescription medications, such as herbs and supplements, and nontraditional therapies, such as acupuncture, massage, or stress reduction.

- Purity: How is it prepared? What other ingredients are included?
- Cost: Is it worth the money involved?

Safety and purity issues are significant, especially for substances taken by mouth. Each brand of a preparation can be made differently, with various stabilizers and purification systems. In contrast to prescription and over-the-counter medications, preparation techniques for supplements are not reviewed for safety by the FDA before being released onto the market. Supplement makers are responsible for ensuring the safety and effectiveness of their products, and these kinds of claims are not evaluated by the federal government before they are sold.

The FDA regulates the safety of the natural supplements, though not their effectiveness for any purpose. All supplements on the market need to be determined as "Generally Recognized As Safe," or GRAS, though no requirements exist to show that a supplement has an effect on any disease or body process.

The FDA describes their role on their Web site (www. foodsafety.gov/~dms/supplmnt.html):

Under the Dietary Supplement Health and Education Act of 1994 (DSHEA), the dietary supplement manufacturer is responsible for ensuring that a dietary supplement is safe before it is marketed. FDA is responsible for taking action against any unsafe dietary supplement product after it reaches the market. Generally, manufacturers do not need to register their products with FDA nor get FDA approval before producing or selling dietary supplements. Manufacturers must make sure that product label information is truthful and not misleading.

As the above statement illustrates, supplement manufacturers do not need FDA approval to market or label their products, and the FDA's responsibility is only to act against unsafe products *after* they reach the market.

In 1997, a purity and labeling issue arose when a product for scalp psoriasis called SkinCap was marketed for nonprescription treatment. This product was manufactured in Spain and later other countries, and sold in the United States as a nonmedication herbal therapy to help psoriasis of the scalp. Many psoriasis sufferers were amazed by the results, and the product became increasingly popular. However, later analysis showed that the manufacturer of SkinCap was surreptitiously adding clobetasol, a super-potent topical steroid, to increase efficacy. This super-potent steroid can be absorbed by the skin into the body, can thin the skin of the scalp, and could potentially react with other steroids being used. When these findings became available, the FDA removed SkinCap from the market. A 2-week study showed that zinc pyrithione spray did not appear to improve the effectiveness of clobetasol foam, so the dramatic effects that were reported may all have been due to the steroid.

Although the majority of products do not contain unlabeled ingredients, it is important to recognize the possibility and investigate what assurances of purity and safety are available.

As medications become available through the Internet and in the global marketplace, it is important to determine where a product comes from and what guarantees exist that a product has ingredients advertised and is manufactured in an appropriate way. Several recent medication contamination cases worldwide highlight the potential risks of mislabeled or improperly manufactured medication.

75. Are there medications that can make psoriasis worse?

Few medicines are known to worsen psoriasis, but any medication or medication changes can affect the skin. In particular, some classes of medications are often reported to worsen psoriasis.

Medications for high blood pressure:

- Thiazide diuretics such as hydrochlorothiazide
- Beta-blockers such as carvedilol, propranolol, labatolol, metoprolol, and acebutolol
- Calcium channel blockers such as nifedepine, amlodipine, verapamil, and diltiazem
- ACE inhibitors such as captopril, enalapril, and lisinopril

Other medications:

- Oral steroids, when reducing/tapering or stopping the dose
- Nonsteroidal anti-inflammatories
- Immunostimulators such as G-CSF, IL-2, interferon-alpha, and interferon-beta
- Antimalarials such as chloroquine, hydroxychloroquine, quinacrine, and quinidine
- Lithium
- In rare reports, glyburide and gemfibrozil

These medications do not cause flares in most people. However, if psoriasis worsens after starting one of these medicines, consider discussing with your doctor

Treatment

whether an alternate medication could be used in its place.

For any medication, if psoriasis worsens after beginning or increasing a dose, consider following the same steps. For new medications, however, such as antibiotics treating an infection, it is important to consider whether the underlying problem might be the trigger for a psoriasis flare.

76. With all of these open areas on the skin, are people with psoriasis at higher risk for infection?

Although it might seem likely that people with psoriasis can easily become infected through open red areas of skin, in most people this is not the case. Psoriasis plaques appear to be protected for several reasons. First, because the skin is rapidly growing and regenerating, skin injuries tend to heal quickly. Second, because there is an increased number of blood vessels bringing nutrients to skin in psoriasis, infections heal quickly. Finally, the large number of immune system cells in the skin that drive psoriasis may help protect from infection as well, if needed.

Unfortunately, people often incorrectly associate the scaly skin of psoriasis with being "dirty."

Because of these protective qualities, skin affected by psoriasis does not need excessive cleaning with antibacterial or alcohol-based products. Gentle cleaning followed by immediate moisturizing with a heavy cream or ointment (discussed in Question 49) is the most effective approach for many people.

Unfortunately, people often incorrectly associate the scaly skin of psoriasis with being "dirty." Trying to treat scaly skin or scalp with aggressive cleaning, such as scrubbing, is unnecessary and can actually make psoriasis worse.

77. Why does healed psoriasis sometimes look darker than healthy skin?

After any trauma to the skin, the skin goes through a healing process. This process involves first restoring the barrier of the skin through healing and then fading and regressing to become a scar. During the second part of this process, healed skin often appears to be a different color, either lighter or darker, than surrounding healthy skin. These color changes may be temporary or may persist for years after the skin surface returns to normal. These changes are called **post-inflammatory changes** and are common to most skin injuries. Many people may observe a change in skin color after a scratch on the arm or the leg, and the same phenomenon can occur when psoriasis heals.

Post-inflammatory changes

Darker or lighter areas of skin that develop after a skin injury, such as psoriasis or an ordinary scrape, resolves.

Although these color changes can be bothersome in healing psoriasis, they tend to decrease or even disappear over time. The appearance of slightly darker or lighter patches of skin is not part of psoriasis but rather the process of healing after psoriasis has resolved. It may be reassuring to know that these pigment changes reflect healing psoriasis and are not seen in active psoriatic skin.

78. I have a special event where I'd like my skin to look its best. What are my options?

While a particular regimen may be effective for controlling psoriasis over time, there are special events in people's lives where they would like to be free of psoriasis. Special events such as a wedding or a landmark anniversary might bring with it hopes for a special day and photographs that will be kept for many years.

If you are planning for a special event in the future, different strategies can help your skin to look its best for the occasion. All of the following approaches require planning ahead and consistent, correct use of medication to be fully effective.

Pulse treatment
The planned use of a very strong or very high-dose medication for a short period of time.

If a person is on low-potency steroids (see potency chart in Table 3) or no steroids, a **pulse treatment** of high-potency topical steroids, or steroid injections into the skin, can cause rapid improvement for a short period. Super-potent steroids are generally approved for use for a 2-week period, and beginning use 2 weeks before an event can help clear the skin. Another way that steroids can be used is by direct injection into psoriatic skin. These injections can be uncomfortable but are generally more effective at reaching the skin when compared to topical formulas. It is important to note that this therapy cannot be continued over a long period without risk of adverse effects. After withdrawing the super-potent steroids the risk of a psoriasis flare is increased and may only be appropriate for limited areas.

Among oral medications, cyclosporine (sold as Neoral or Sandimmune), oral tacrolimus (sold as ProGraf), or methotrexate can be started before a special event is planned. Cyclosporine is probably the fastest, but planning several months in advance is recommended. Some people need these drugs all the time to control psoriasis, but they are also appropriate to use for a short period of time. Like super-potent topical steroids, with oral medications there is a risk of side effects and flare after the treatment is stopped.

Biologic therapies can be effective for short-term use and rapid response. Of the biologic therapies currently in use, infliximab appears to have the most rapid onset, but all biologics can be used successfully with appropriate planning.

Each of these and other approaches to short-term improvement of psoriasis has potential benefits and real risks. A serious discussion with your physician about your short- and long-term treatment goals is essential before beginning any short-term therapy increase.

79. What happens if I stop taking my medications?

When treatment is stopped, some people may stay in remission, some may relapse back to their original condition, and some can **rebound** and have the psoriasis reappear more severely than before. Whether this happens depends on both the person and the medications being used. The National Psoriasis Foundation and many research studies formally define rebound in a specific way. Rebound in these situations occurs when psoriasis becomes 25% worse than baseline levels (discussed in Question 72) or when psoriasis changes from plaque type to a more severe type such as pustular or erythrodermic psoriasis.

When stopping any medication being taken for psoriasis, the best way to prevent rebound is to consult with your physician so you understand whether it should be stopped abruptly, discontinued slowly, or changed gradually to something else. Some medications used generally for other reasons, such as oral steroids, are known to provoke rebound flares and must be monitored carefully if discontinued.

Rebound

In psoriasis, a rapid worsening of skin disease; typically the psoriasis worsens beyond its original severity after a medication is stopped.

Jason's comment:

It can be difficult to manage the timing of prescription refills, but it's important. My psoriasis flared from missing just a few days of treatment, and it took me weeks to get back to where I had been.

80. Which treatments can be used during pregnancy?

A woman with psoriasis considering pregnancy should consult with a dermatologist and/or an obstetrician to ensure that none of her medications interferes with conception or pregnancy. Even using medications that have reasonably safe profiles is a very personal decision and may require a specific consultation. Because most medications aren't tested directly in pregnant women, there will always be areas in which the effects are unknown.

People with mild psoriasis can usually control their disease safely with topical medicines.

People with mild psoriasis can usually control their disease safely with topical medicines. While topical medicines have fewer side effects than oral medicines, they can absorb through the skin and into the blood. This is especially true for medicines that are used frequently or over a large area of the body. Super-potent steroids and vitamin A derivatives such as tazarotene can be absorbed into the blood, and could potentially cause problems in pregnancy. After birth, many oral medications can pass into breast milk (discussed in Question 81).

Although some topical medications can be absorbed into the body, the greatest pregnancy risks come from using systemic medications. These systemic therapies can last in the body for months, even after they are stopped.

Methotrexate is the only medication known to affect sperm. Men using methotrexate are advised to wait 6 months after stopping the medication to try for conception.

Medications that persist in the body include the oral vitamin A derivatives acitretin, isotretinoin, and tazarotene, and the folate antagonist methotrexate. Women on these medications must plan to stop these medications months to years before a pregnancy or may wish to avoid them altogether until after having a family. Among these medications, tazarotene and methotrexate leave the body after one menstrual cycle, while acitretin (sold as Soriatane) can persist in the body for up to 3 years and is generally not used in women of child-bearing potential.

Many women find that their psoriasis improves during pregnancy. The normal mild immune suppression seen during pregnancy that protects a baby also decreases the severity of psoriasis and many other immune-mediated diseases. However, during pregnancy the response to treatment is unpredictable, and some women will need to adjust their medication. If psoriasis is severe, a woman may want to stabilize the disease with medications that are relatively safe during pregnancy before trying to get pregnant. All women who want to become pregnant should practice good prenatal care and nutrition, including taking a multivitamin and folate supplement to reduce the chance of a birth defect.

All prescription medications have a package insert indicating whether they are safe for use in pregnancy. Drugs are classified into risk categories by the FDA (**Table 8**). The categories for commonly used psoriasis medications are shown in **Table 9**. Of note, many of

131

Table 8   FDA Drug Classification Categories

Drug Risk Category	Definition
A	Controlled studies show no fetal risk
B	No risk to human fetus despite possible animal risk; or no risk in animal studies and human studies have not been done
C	Risk cannot be ruled out; human studies are lacking Animal studies may or may not show risk Potential benefits may justify potential risk
D	Positive evidence for risk to human fetus, however, benefits may outweigh risks of the drug
X	Contraindicated in pregnancy; drug should not be used during pregnancy
Unrated	No pregnancy category has been assigned

the biologics are category B and may be of value to people with severe psoriasis or psoriatic arthritis during their pregnancy.

Other resources for drugs safe during pregnancy include the American Academy of Pediatrics (www.aap.org) and your doctor or health plan. Ultimately, all treatment decisions during pregnancy should be made with the input of your doctor.

81. Which treatments can be used while breastfeeding?

When evaluating medication safety when breastfeeding, it is useful to consider the similarities and differences between pregnancy and breastfeeding for medications. During pregnancy, drugs can pass from mother to baby via the placenta, whereas during breastfeeding, babies can receive medication through breast milk. Of course, the benefits of breastfeeding for the infant vs. risks of absorbtion vs. comfort and well-being of the mother have to be weighed thoughtfully.

Direct studies are not always performed to determine whether medications pass into breast milk, so information

Table 9   Medications Commonly Used in Psoriasis

Type of Medication	Pregnancy Category
Topical	
Steroids	C
Calcipotriene/calcipotriol	C
Tazarotene	X
Tacrolimus/pimecrolimus	C
Light Therapies	
Sunlight	B
UVB	B
Psoralen + UVA	X
Oral Medications	
Methotrexate	X
Cyclosporine	C
Tacrolimus	C
Acitretin (Soriatane)	X
Tazarotene	X
Biologic Therapies	
Infliximab (Remicade)	B
Etanercept (Enbrel)	B
Alefacept (Amevive)	B
Adalimumab (Humira)	B
Golimumab (Simponi)	B
Ustekinumab (Stellara)	B

about breastfeeding is often incomplete. This is especially true for newer medications such as biologic therapies, which are rarely given to lactating women.

Lists of drugs that are known to be safe for breastfeeding women, as well as those that are recommended to be used with caution, are available. Among drugs for psoriasis, recommendations for the following medications are available from the American Academy of Pediatrics Policy Statement (www.aap.org):

- Usually compatible with breastfeeding: Acetaminophen, ibuprofen for joint pain
- Caution when using: Sulfasalazine
- Not safe for use: Methotrexate, cyclosporine

It's unlikely that most biologics that are excreted into breast milk are absorbed by breastfeeding infants because the molecules are very susceptible to digestion, which is why they can't be given orally. Nonetheless, there is very limited information about women who have chosen to breastfeed under these circumstances.

Web sites that can offer more information include:

- www.aap.org/healthtopics/breastfeeding.cfm
- World Health Organization Recommendations, 2002 (www.who.int/child-adolescent-health/New_ Publications/NUTRITION/BF_Maternal_ Medication.pdf)

PART FIVE

Social Effects of Psoriasis

I don't have health insurance. How can I get care for my psoriasis?

What are common problems faced by people with psoriasis?

What are some of the ways people deal with their psoriasis? How do I cope with knowing I have psoriasis?

More . . .

82. I don't have health insurance. How can I get care for my psoriasis?

Carla's comment:

Here are my suggestions if you don't have medical insurance and you need to care for your psoriasis:

1. *Research dermatology schools or institutes that offer clinical trials on the different medications of psoriasis.*
2. *Research the library, Internet, publications, etc. for "natural remedies" to psoriasis, such as suggestions on what type of food to eat, what vitamins to take, etc.*
3. *Take up yoga or meditation to help control stress levels.*
4. *Use over-the-counter psoriasis medicines, oils, lotions, etc. There are quite a few that help control the itching, such as Neutrogena T-Gel, petroleum jelly, Cetaphil lotion, and so on.*

Depending on the severity of your disease, options include local free clinics staffed by volunteer physicians or a free treatment day at a local medical school. Unfortunately, no single resource is available that can help find dermatologic care for the uninsured in every geographic area. Clinical trials can offer some short- and medium-term treatment options. Some foundations working with drug companies or the companies themselves will offer assistance for medication to low-income patients.

For someone with psoriasis, health insurance coverage is very useful and important.

For someone with psoriasis, health insurance coverage is very useful and important. Consider investigating options for coverage such as purchasing through work or with a cooperative purchasing group. When leaving a job for most reasons, workers and their families have the option of purchasing equivalent coverage through COBRA (a federal law called the Consolidated

Omnibus Reconciliation Act) provisions within the first 90 days, though the worker is responsible for the cost. Most cities and states have subsidized health plans that help uninsured individuals buy insurance; these will vary by location. Most children are eligible for health care through CHIP, the Children's Health Insurance Plan, which is mandated by the federal government and administered by individual states.

People with disabling psoriasis may be eligible for short- or long-term disability support. The application for health insurance coverage, whether through work, the government, or other means, can be lengthy and complicated. Although it can be cumbersome, the process of identifying and securing health coverage is important for people with psoriasis.

83. What are common problems faced by people with psoriasis?

Sue's comment:

I mastered wearing clothes that would not reveal my skin condition to my co-workers because I was so embarrassed at how awful it looked. Most of my co-workers were completely unaware of my condition. One of my bosses was getting more and more skeptical about my going to so many medical appointments and was suggesting that I was faking it. I finally took her into an office and undressed. She never questioned me again about my illness.

Jason's comment:

During my worst stretches, I was embarrassed about the several band-aids I wore on each hand—not for appearance but because my knuckles were cracking. Looking back, I am amazed by how understanding my co-workers were, but if it got that bad again I know I would be just as self-conscious.

People with psoriasis face many common problems, beginning with the challenge of having a "public" skin disease. Unlike kidney disease or diabetes, for example, psoriasis may be difficult or impossible to conceal. Unfortunately, the appearance of skin diseases such as psoriasis can diminish the privacy enjoyed by most people regarding their medical conditions.

As a result of this "public appearance," people with psoriasis might be stared at or questioned, unlike someone with an "invisible" medical problem. Some people may jump to conclusions about psoriasis and might incorrectly believe that skin and scalp scaling is a result of too little cleaning. As a result, a person with psoriasis might find himself or herself explaining the disease to strangers—an important public service but tiring as well.

In everyday life, during hobbies and vacations, psoriasis can limit what a person chooses to wear. Shorts? A short-sleeve shirt? A bathing suit? The appearance of psoriasis in public can cause anxiety. Interestingly, most people find that when they begin to ignore feelings of self-consciousness and wear what they choose, they feel happier and freer to do what they like. Ignoring your psoriasis and doing anything you choose for a weekend or a vacation might be worth a try.

In romantic relationships, as well, psoriasis can feel burdensome. It might be the symptoms of psoriasis itself or simply the negative feelings associated with its appearance that affect interpersonal relationships. Sometimes a person's negative thoughts and feelings about psoriasis can be far worse than their physical disease, and can feel like an unbearable burden. It might help to think of psoriasis as a skin disease, no more or less, that bears no reflection on who a person is. Talking to others who have experienced these feelings can help lessen the loneliness and may help with finding solutions that work for you.

John's comment:

I let my latest boss know up front that I have psoriasis, after I got the job. By letting him know that I have psoriasis, if he notices some of my psoriasis I hope he would at least know that it isn't contagious. In order to alleviate possible questioning about whether I really have as many doctor appointments as I have, I copy my boss on my doctor referral requests sent to my primary care physician's office.

84. How do people usually feel about psoriasis?

Sue's comment:

I know that there are differences in the way people experience psoriasis. I had fairly small plaques but they were all over my body (about 80% of my surface area): in my ears, under my breasts, larger plaques on my back, my abdomen, and on my buttocks, but these most people never saw because they were typically under my clothing. It completely covered my scalp. I had no psoriasis on my face.

I hated how painful it was. I could not comfortably wear a brassiere. It was difficult to sit. I was always aware of how messy it was. There were flakes everywhere in my car, on my desk at work, at conference tables when I was in meetings. I used to measure the flakes in my bed in the morning. Three tablespoons a day. My skin would crack and bleed through my clothes.

Some people with psoriasis feel incredibly dismayed with their disease, while others consider it a small part of their life. Although psoriasis doesn't cause life-threatening

Some people with psoriasis feel incredibly dismayed with their disease, while others consider it a small part of their life.

symptoms for most people, its affect on an individual's life and the daily limitations are often underestimated. In particular, sufferers report wanting to hide their disease, limitations on wearing short sleeves and shorts, and worries in interpersonal relationships.

A new body of research is emerging that is based on understanding the impact of psoriasis and other diseases on people's daily life. Surveys that measure the quality of life and degrees of unhappiness among patients show a striking level of unhappiness because of psoriasis. Self-reported quality of life was considered worse for someone with psoriasis than for someone with heart disease after a heart attack. Over time, psoriasis can even cause a psychological burden on par with kidney failure.

Physicians and patients recognize that the goal of treatment is to improve quality of life, in addition to minimizing skin changes.

John's comment:

When my psoriasis is active on or behind my ears I am very self-conscious when I go for a hair cut. However, on one such visit, the person cutting my hair was very kind. She said, "Oh you have psoriasis," and then proceeded to explain that one of her relatives had it and she cuts that person's hair. Although this is a very rare interaction, it was heartening.

85. What are some of the ways people deal with their psoriasis? How do I cope with knowing I have psoriasis?

Carolyn's comment:

When I was younger I had psoriasis mostly just on my scalp, so it was easier to conceal. I remember seeing patches on my mom's face near the eyebrows and nose. She didn't

seem too concerned about it. She did put medicated oint-
ments on it, but she didn't seem self-conscious about it. Per-
haps my mother's attitude helped me cope with it better
when my psoriasis started appearing on my legs and arms
and other obvious places. To cope with these areas, I did
wear pants more than skirts and shorts. But I didn't let it
stop me from wearing a bathing suit or shorts when the
weather called for it. The best way to deal with it is to just
answer people honestly when asked about what it is. It's
not much different than having freckles or red hair, once
you get past a few encounters with curious people.

From the time of first diagnosis to years of living with
psoriasis, people find many different ways to deal with
their skin disease and its effects on their lifestyle. Several different approaches may be effective; it might help
to try a different approach at different times in your life.

- Learn as much as you can.
  Becoming well educated about psoriasis can help
  prepare you for the future and the therapeutic decisions you will make with your doctor. Because no
  one treatment can cure psoriasis, understanding the
  benefits and risks of all your options is essential for
  developing a treatment plan.
- Be proactive with your treatment plan.
  Finding a physician you trust to help treat your psoriasis is essential. A physician who you can speak
  with comfortably and openly, in addition to having
  experience and expertise, can help alleviate many
  common worries. Make sure you understand your
  treatments and that your doctor is able to answer
  your questions.
- Communicate with friends and family.
  Being as open and honest as you can with family and
  friends will help them to understand your disease and

may relieve some of the stress that comes from feeling alone. Explaining psoriasis can demystify the skin disease, and asking for help when you need it can help you stay connected with those close to you. Often, many people want to help friends and significant others with psoriasis or any disease but don't know how. Asking for specific support, such as putting lotion on a hard-to-reach place or planning a vacation somewhere sunny, can be very helpful to them as well.

- Meet other people with psoriasis.

One common complaint shared by many people with psoriasis is that they feel alone. Connecting with other people who have similar experiences can be comforting and fun, and can yield useful suggestions. The National Psoriasis Foundation has several formats, including a message board and information about support groups, for people with psoriasis. Their annual nationwide patient and physician meeting is another opportunity to meet people and learn more about psoriasis (see Appendix for more information).

- Have a sense of humor.

As challenging as it can seem, keeping a sense of humor about life and your experiences can help alleviate stress and bring perspective to the serious business of staying healthy.

One common complaint shared by many people with psoriasis is that they feel alone.

86. Are there support groups for people with psoriasis? How do I find out about them?

Both national and local groups exist for psoriasis sufferers to meet and communicate. Subjects range from treatment options, to medical information and research, to everyday life with psoriasis. The National Psoriasis Foundation hosts many such groups and does an especially good job of working to connect children and teens with psoriasis. Many energetic people host information sites on the Internet and often plan meetings in different areas. Internet chat, bulletin boards, and even pen-pal matching services are available for people who'd like to connect with others.

At the national level, the National Psoriasis Foundation hosts an annual meeting each year at different locations around the country. Attendees rave about both the wealth of information available as well as the opportunity to connect with people from all over the country. The opportunity to "take a break" from being the only person with psoriasis and be surrounded by others who share similar challenges can be relaxing and energizing.

For children and teens, summer programs exist for kids with psoriasis and other skin diseases (see the Appendix). These "sleep-away camps" are usually 1 to 2 weeks long and are supervised by both counselors and dermatologists. Most are free or subsidized by sponsoring organizations. For many children, this is a unique opportunity to spend a week without standing out because of their skin.

87. I just found out that I have psoriasis and I feel depressed. Is this common?

Carla's comment:

It took awhile before I accepted that I have psoriasis. I saw more than a dozen physicians and dermatologists. In the beginning the diagnosis varied from eczema, ringworm, mosquito bite, and so on. But when I lived in a cold climate for a few months and my psoriasis increased, the diagnosis of several doctors all pointed to psoriasis. I became depressed when I found out there was not a cure for this. I also became depressed when I found out there was no one in my family who had this. I was the first one. The depression comes and goes, and it could occur in either major situations (such as new psoriasis plaques appearing) or minor situations (such as being too ashamed to wear outfits that will expose the plaques). I don't think the feelings of depression will go away, but in time I was able to minimize the length of time I felt depressed.

The diagnosis of psoriasis may come as a surprise and can be a relief for someone trying to understand a chronic skin disease. The news of its chronic, lifelong nature can be worrisome and saddening. It can be normal to initially retreat from everyday life as you begin to gather information and understand the implications of psoriasis and its treatment. Some may feel self-conscious or embarrassed about psoriatic skin, which can lead to depression, a fear of rejection, social isolation, or worries about intimacy.

Because psoriasis affects many young people, psoriasis is often their first experience with a disease that is not immediately curable.

Some feel socially isolated—as if they're being punished with a chronic disease, dismayed with the lack of control they have over this aspect of their health, or angry at unexpected and unwanted news. Because psoriasis affects many young people, psoriasis is often their first experience with a disease that is not immediately curable. All of these reactions are normal.

At times, you might feel withdrawn, lose interest in everyday activities that used to be enjoyable, change sleeping and eating patterns, or cry often for days or weeks. It is possible that a more severe form of depression is developing; professional help may be warranted.

It is important to recognize that the diagnosis of psoriasis, like that of any chronic disease, is usually unexpected and can be very saddening. Sadness, anger, denial, or withdrawal can all occur as part of a normal response. Over time, most people come to an understanding and acceptance of psoriasis.

88. How does the diagnosis of psoriasis affect me, my partner, and our relationship?

Carla's comment:

For those who know that I have psoriasis, I am fortunate enough to experience acceptance. My family, friends, and personal relationships have made me feel that they can see past the psoriasis and treat me normally. The initial reaction is usually curiosity about what causes this disease. Some have even become as passionate as I am in finding a cure. Since the time I had psoriasis, I can count on one hand the number of people who have seen my psoriasis. The ones who don't know still don't have a clue until today that I have it, and I may add, it takes a tremendous amount of time and effort to hide it.

A new diagnosis of psoriasis, like that of any chronic disease, requires adjustments in daily routines and may even change the way people think about themselves. Like most things in life, the way a person thinks about psoriasis can change greatly over time. A partner's understanding of psoriasis—what it is, what causes it, that it's not contagious—is an important part of the relationship.

When a person is first diagnosed, surprise, dismay, and frustration are common. An individual may look to his or her partner for reassurance and support during this time. A partner's commitment of support and understanding can go a long way toward alleviating a patient's worries about the skin disease. Your partner may worry about the effect of his or her skin's appearance on intimacy. Touching your partner, even for a hug, can help alleviate these concerns.

Over time, people with psoriasis develop ways to live well with their disease. They may or may not look to people in their lives for emotional support and physical help (applying cream or lotion, for example), so it can be helpful to offer help, and then let the other person ask for help as needed. As a partner, your presence, support, and reassurance can be invaluable to a person who has recently been diagnosed with a disease. As a person with psoriasis, your partner may want to help, but may not be sure how to start. Asking for help when needed allows your partner to participate in your life in a meaningful way.

For both partners, open communication is challenging but essential. Both people may be going through an adjustment process for months or even years. Activities and routines may need to be redefined, especially if a person has psoriatic arthritis. Although the process can be challenging, it can result in strengthened lines of communication.

89. Is it okay to have intimate contact with a partner if I have psoriasis?

Absolutely—there is no physical reason why a person with psoriasis can't have intimate contact with his or her partner. Women on certain oral medications for psoriasis need to avoid becoming pregnant; however, there is no need to limit sexual activity with the proper precautions. One caution is to postpone sexual activity when psoriasis causes raw, painful skin on the genitals.

Although there are few physical limitations preventing intimate contact, many patients describe how their psoriasis negatively affects their sexual relationships. It is important to recognize that psoriasis, like any disease, can cause a person to feel isolated, self-conscious, or less sexually attractive. These feelings can lead to decreased interest in sex. Over time, people adjust to life with psoriasis and feel like their "normal" selves in life and in relationships.

Although it can be challenging at times, keeping communication open with a partner is critical to dispel misconceptions and alleviate fears. The key is talking to relieve any concerns and finding an accepting and understanding partner.

Fortunately, intimate contact doesn't have to be limited to intercourse. Touching, caring, and pleasure are all important. Physical intimacy can be guided by the desires of both partners at a given time. For most relationships, close physical contact can be a reassuring and happy way to spend time together when a person feels different about his or her body due to psoriasis.

Fortunately, intimate contact doesn't have to be limited to intercourse.

90. Someone close to me was recently diagnosed with psoriasis. What can I do to help?

Carolyn's comment:

Just talking with someone who has psoriasis, asking questions, and showing interest is helpful, both to you and your friend who has been diagnosed. Friends have helped me by learning more and encouraging me to learn more, especially as new treatments have become available. Friends of mine have sent me information leads on the Internet.

The support of friends and family is incredibly valuable to a person adjusting to a new diagnosis of psoriasis.

As a friend, reassurance of your presence and support may be all that is needed. This includes taking time to listen, affirming your friend's feelings, and being available over time. Different people need a different amount or type of help, so help can simply consist of being available and responding to their requests. Continue doing the activities you have enjoyed doing together or, if that person isn't able to continue the same activities, establish new traditions.

If a friend is anxious about psoriasis, take time to listen. Avoid minimizing your friend's feelings ("It's really not that bad."), and acknowledge how psoriasis could affect these feelings. Comparisons to other diseases, such as, "At least it's not cancer," are less useful. While people rarely die from psoriasis, it can cause extreme emotional distress, and it can take time to adjust to this permanent change in their skin. If a friend shows signs of serious depression after being diagnosed with psoriasis—a depressed mood, a loss of interest in activities, changes in eating or sleeping patterns, loss of energy, feeling worthless or guilty, lack of concentration, or thoughts of death—encourage him or her to seek professional help.

Because people newly diagnosed with psoriasis can feel isolated and alone, the presence of friends and loved ones through this process is a crucial part of the support they may need.

91. How do people talk about their psoriasis with others?

Carolyn's comment:

Talking with people about psoriasis is always an interesting experience. In summertime people have made comments or questions, ranging from asking if I had blackfly bites to ask-ing if I had run into poison oak or poison ivy. I always answer honestly that I have psoriasis, which I think proba-bly assures people that it is not something contagious. I have had young children ask me what I have on my skin—kids are always so open and honest with their questions. I usu-ally try to explain it to them in simple terms. Not too many children have seen the old ads about "the heartbreak of pso-riasis" or know what the word is. So I tell them it is a skin problem, that it itches, and that they can't catch it.

Depending on the crowd, people around you may know a lot or next to nothing about psoriasis. Learning to explain it briefly can save time and questions for you.

People's curiosity may range from simply, "What is that?" to more complex worries like, "Is this conta-gious?" Fortunately these questions can be anticipated and are easily answered. Especially for children, who tend to be curious, a quick and no-nonsense explana-tion of skin disease can help to demystify the subject.

When first diagnosed with psoriasis, some people pre-fer to hide their disease under long-sleeve clothing, long pants, or a hat. Over time, however, many people with psoriasis find that a short explanation to others allows them to wear what they please and continue with the activities of daily life. Much of the discomfort of other people around psoriasis may stem from curi-ous looks, and explaining the basics of the disease—that it's immune-mediated, chronic, not infectious, and not contagious—can quickly quell those stares.

When learning about something new, listeners usually take cues from the person who is explaining. Some people find that when they present psoriasis in a

When learning about something new, listeners usually take cues from the person who is explaining.

matter-of-fact way, or as "not a big deal," other people will think about it in the same way.

Trial and error may be the most effective way to develop good communication about psoriasis. The National Psoriasis Foundation has more resources and message boards for those interested in talking about psoriasis with others.

John's comment:

After 20+ years I am more likely to mention it in conversation with close friends or close associates.

92. Will psoriasis affect the jobs I can do?

For the majority of people with mild psoriasis, the answer will be a qualified "No." Nonetheless, psoriasis can cause challenges at work. These issues may range from general discomfort and itching to self-consciousness about a flaky scalp (no doubt reinforced by advertisements for antidandruff shampoos) to the desire to cover up. Compounding the problem is the fact that psoriasis can cause days of missed work, require time for treatment, and can be very costly due to over-the-counter therapies.

People with scalp psoriasis may have to overcome the appearance of scales that look like dandruff on dark clothing and suits. Unfortunately, the appearance of skin flakes may be incorrectly associated by some people with inadequate showering or a lack of cleanliness. Heightened awareness of the disease can help dispel these myths.

People who have felt professionally limited include a swimming coach who didn't want to get in the pool in front of his team and a teacher afraid to wear short sleeves and reveal her elbows around her students. Many daily activities at work and in personal life can be affected by psoriasis. Some of these limitations can be overcome by educating co-workers about the disease; it is up to each individual to decide what he or she feels comfortable doing.

Severe hand and foot psoriasis, moderate-to-severe psoriasis, and psoriatic arthritis can often pose significant work limitations. People with severe arthritis of any cause may need accommodations in terms of responsibilities or work schedules, sometimes leading in extreme cases to the need for disability. Proactive treatment of joint disease and planning with a supervisor for jobs that a person can continue to do will help those with severe arthritis to remain in the workforce.

John's comment:

It is my belief that some people's judgments in the workplace are significantly influenced by physical appearance, and hence being able to treat psoriasis that is evident can be important for purposes of one's job. Other aspects of psoriasis that can affect work can include pain, flaking, itching, bleeding, time needed for treatment, or doctor appointments.

93. Does stress affect psoriasis?

Carolyn's comment:

I believe stress does affect psoriasis—it increases the symptoms. I used to fantasize that the perfect solution for psoriasis would be to teach sailing on some subtropical island. Low stress and good sun and lots of salt water. I had my skin clear up completely on a 6-week trip through the South Pacific.

Stress can clearly play a role in psoriasis and many other immune-mediated diseases, including lupus and multiple sclerosis. The word "stress" encompasses both physical and emotional triggers, and recent research has sought to understand how identifying and minimizing these influences can improve immune-mediated disease.

Stresses that have been shown in formal studies to be associated with worsening immune-mediated diseases are shown in **Table 10**.

Emotional stress from life events can be short-term (**acute**) or chronic and has been shown to exacerbate many immune diseases as well. Stress can be triggered by a number of life changes, whether they are unhappy or happy ones. The various life events listed below have been found (by Holmes in 1967, while developing the commonly used Social Readjustment Scale) to cause the most stress in people's lives.

Life changes that cause severe stress include:

- Spouse or partner's death
- Divorce
- Marital separation
- Jail term
- Death of close family member
- Marriage
- Fired from work
- Marital reconciliation
- Retirement
- Change in health of a family member
- Pregnancy

A relaxing time, such as a vacation, can cause skin improvement for many people with psoriasis. The effectiveness of many treatment plans, such as the

Acute

Refers to immediate or short-term changes, usually within hours or days.

Table 10   Stresses and the Immune-Mediated Diseases That They Are Reported to Worsen

Physical Stress Factor	Disease
Infection	Psoriasis, lupus, dermatitis
Change in medications	Psoriasis, psoriatic arthritis, lupus, and pemphigus
Dramatic change in diet	Pemphigus
Heat exposure	Pemphigus
Childbirth	Grave's disease, Hashimoto's thyroiditis
Menstruation	Myasthenia gravis
Alcohol intoxication (binge drinking)	Psoriasis
Sunburn	Dermatitis, pemphigus
Traumatic injury	Multiple sclerosis

Goeckerman regimen, which involves several weeks in the hospital, is thought to be due in part to limiting the stress of daily life. Treatment with salt water and sun at the Dead Sea also appears to have significant beneficial effects. Stress reduction has a clearly beneficial role in therapy for many immune-mediated diseases such as psoriasis. The relative role of stress on skin disease for any given person is variable.

Although it is virtually impossible to avoid stress in daily life, routines and habits that minimize stress can be helpful for psoriasis and overall health.

Stress reduction has a clearly beneficial role in therapy for many immune-mediated diseases such as psoriasis.

94. Do pregnancy and menopause improve or worsen psoriasis symptoms?

Pregnancy sometimes makes psoriasis better, but the effects of changing hormones in the body seem to vary considerably in different people. Unfortunately, some women who improve during pregnancy will get worse after their baby is born. Menopause can make psoriasis worse, and often makes the skin drier, which can make it more vulnerable to outbreaks. A severe form of psoriasis—generalized pustular psoriasis—can be

provoked by premenstrual hormonal changes, by pregnancy, and by high-dose estrogen therapy, though fortunately this last problem is rare.

95. Do drinking alcohol and smoking affect psoriasis?

Alcoholism and alcohol misuse are more common in
people with psoriasis than in the general population. This
finding may be related to the emotional burden of having
a stigmatizing disease. Alcohol use appears to worsen the
disease, and abstinence alone has been reported to lead to
remission in some people. Similarly, restarting drinking
can be associated with psoriasis recurrence.

Cigarette smoking and tobacco use are more common
among psoriasis patients than in the general population and have been noted by some researchers to contribute to the development of pustular psoriasis.
However, smoking is also common among those who
misuse alcohol, a fact that can confuse the issue.
Although older studies could not conclusively link
smoking to worsening psoriasis, some newer data suggest that people who smoke are more likely to have
worse cases of psoriasis. It is not yet clear whether
smoking itself makes psoriasis worse or if it is simply a
consequence of an individual's attempt to relieve stress
due to worsening psoriasis. Regardless of the role of
cause and effect in smoking and psoriasis, it is clear
that stopping smoking has incredible health benefits.

96. Does the weather or the temperature affect psoriasis?

Carla's comment:

*In the 8 years I have had psoriasis, I am able to conclude
that the cold weather (55 degrees and below) triggers the*

plaques [to] increase and appear more often. A humid, warm climate is really good for my psoriasis. I rarely put medicine on when I am in this kind of climate.

The weather, especially different seasons, does affect psoriasis in most people. The increased sunlight in spring and summer can improve psoriasis, and the decreased sun in fall and winter (especially in northern latitudes) can worsen it. Over time, most people can tell whether their psoriasis is responsive to sunlight.

The potentially beneficial effects of weather and temperature on psoriasis make certain destinations therapeutic for psoriasis. Some people find that the ocean or salty bodies of water, such as the Dead Sea, help psoriatic skin. The relative contribution of the water, the hot, dry temperatures, and the sunny weather isn't clear, but these conditions seem to be effective.

Weather and temperature therapy for psoriasis is sometimes called **climatotherapy**—therapy involving a specific climate. Sunlight therapy is formally referred to as **heliotherapy**, which means "using the sun." Some locations such as the Dead Sea offer vacation packages that incorporate therapeutic bathing with sightseeing and vacation time.

97. Many treatments on the Internet claim to heal psoriasis. How do I evaluate these claims?

Determining the quality of information among the thousands of web pages on the Internet can be a daunting task for any expert. Each Web site is arranged differently, with descriptions of a product, its effects,

Climatotherapy
Treatment of psoriasis by going to a climate that is likely to improve psoriasis due to the sunlight exposure and sometimes humidity.

Heliotherapy
Treatment of psoriasis by going to a climate that is likely to improve psoriasis due to sunlight exposure.

and information supporting the claim. A few guidelines can help with initial evaluation:

- What is the evidence backing up a claim? Phrases such as "clinical trials" usually describe studies in people, whereas phrases such as "data" or "information" are less specific and harder to evaluate. Does the evidence describe studies in a particular number of people or consist only of testimonials from individuals who rave about a product? Has the product been tested in humans or only in the laboratory?
- Does the web site have a medical advisory board that reviews and evaluates information on the site? Who is on the medical board of a particular web site? Look for sites that are reviewed by expert physicians in a particular field, such as dermatology, rheumatology (joint diseases and immune diseases), or pharmacology.
- Is there published research that backs up these claims? If so, where was this research carried out? Research published by government organizations such as the **National Institutes of Health (NIH)** or university hospitals may be more objectively presented than research done internally by a product's manufacturer.
- Is a therapy marketed as a prescription drug or as a **nutritional supplement**? Although neither category of therapy is guaranteed to be beneficial in a given patient, FDA approval for prescription drugs requires a certain set of standards for effectiveness prior to use. Manufacturers of nutritional supplements are not required to prove effectiveness before marketing a product.
- For an herbal supplement, look for the names of active ingredients (the ingredients thought to be responsible for the beneficial effects of the therapy).

National Institutes of Health (NIH)

The National Institutes of Health is the primary center for medical research in the United States, as well as one of the world's leading research centers. It is the agency within the Department of Health and Human Services responsible for most of its medical research programs and related functions, including the National Library of Medicine.

Nutritional supplement

As defined by the FDA, a nutritional supplement is a product intended to supplement the diet that contains one or more of the following dietary ingredients: a vitamin, a mineral, an herb or other botanical, an amino acid, or a dietary substance to supplement the diet by increasing the total daily intake.

Evaluation of these ingredients is important to identify potential beneficial effects, side effects, and drug interactions before use.

All information about a disease or treatment should be considered in the context of a particular person's illness. Consider discussing new treatments of all types with your doctor. Especially if you have psoriasis and another illness such as diabetes, or are taking multiple medications, careful evaluation of claims before use can prevent unwanted side effects and drug interactions.

98. Are there famous people who have psoriasis?

Psoriasis inflicts all types of people. Famous individuals who most likely had psoriasis include:

- LeAnn Rimes, Grammy Award winning country singer
- John Updike, American novelist and short-story writer
- Vladimir Nabokov, Russian author of many classics, including *Lolita*
- Joseph Stalin, dictator of the Soviet Union during World War II
- Art Garfunkel, musician
- Jerry Mathers, actor, star of "Leave it to Beaver"
- Tom Robbins, American author
- Kenneth Starr, special prosecutor
- CariDee English, "America's Next Top Model" winner in season 7
- Janis Byron, a British pianist with psoriatic arthritis of the fingers
- Abimael Guzman, leader of the guerilla movement, Shining Path, in Peru

- Robert Bruce, King of Scotland from 1274 to 1329, and the father of William Wallace of "Braveheart" fame

Despite how common psoriasis is, few current celebrities or high-profile individuals speak openly about personal experiences with this skin disease. As a result, general awareness about psoriasis may not be as high as for other diseases or cancer.

99. How is psoriasis portrayed in the movies?

There are several movies that have portrayed psoriasis on the big screen. Examples of movies in which psoriasis is involved in the plot include:

- "The Singing Detective" (2003)
  Robert Downey, Jr. stars as a crime novelist suffering from extreme psoriasis and arthritis. The movie was written by accomplished British television writer Dennis Potter and deals honestly with his experience with skin disease and the treatment side effects of psoriasis. Mr. Potter has severe psoriasis and psoriatic arthritis. Interestingly, the conclusion of the movie describes his psoriasis disappearing when he works through personal problems, an optimistic but probably unrealistic ending.
- "Midway" (1976)
  Robert Mitchum stars as Admiral Bull Halsey in this dramatization of the events in the Pacific theater during World War II. The story is loosely based on historical events, when the admiral experiences a psoriasis flare during the Battle of Midway.

A fascinating and entertaining web site hosted by the University of California, San Francisco, shows many different skin diseases in the media at www.skinema.com.

Along with an impressive archive of photos, the web site discusses the accuracies and inaccuracies about skin disease as seen in the entertainment industry.

100. Where can I find more information?

As a patient, caregiver, or family member, you may have specific questions, want to contact others with psoriasis, or find a specialist. The Appendix that follows offers resources.

Organizations

The National Psoriasis Foundation
6600 SW 92nd Ave.
Suite 300
Portland, OR 97223-7195
(503) 244-7404
(800) 723-9166
Fax: (503) 245-0626
e-mail: *getinfo@psoriasis.org*
http://www.psoriasis.org

The American Academy of Dermatology
PO Box 4014
Schaumburg, IL 60168-4014
(847) 330-0230
Fax: (847) 330-0050
http://www.aad.org
http://www.skincarephysicians.com/psoriasisnet

The Food and Drug Administration
http://www.fda.gov
Lists all drugs currently approved by the FDA.
http://www.accessdata.fda.gov/scripts/cder/drugsatfda/index.cfm

Finding a Dermatologist

The American Academy of Dermatology
http://www.aad.org
Click on "Find a Dermatologist." This feature allows you to search for a dermatologist by zip code.

The National Psoriasis Foundation
http://www.psoriasis.org/netcommunity/learn_doctordirectory

American Medical Association
http://www.ama-assn.org
You have the option to select a physician through the "Doctor Finder" feature. Physicians are listed by specialty and by location. Your health plan's directory of participating dermatologists. Dermatologists are often found under specialty listings in the directory.

Clinical Research Resources

Clinical Trials
http://www.clinicaltrials.gov
An online registry of all federally and privately supported ongoing clinical trials conducted in the United States and most from around the world.

Centerwatch
http://www.centerwatch.com
An online listing of worldwide clinical trials recruiting patients with optional e-mail notification about new trials.

Supplements and Complementary Therapies

The Food and Drug Administration
http://vm.cfsan.fda.gov/~dms/ds-savvy.html

United States Pharmacopeia
http://www.usp.org/USPVerified/dietarySupplements
USP is a non-governmental, nonprofit, standard-setting authority for medications and supplements sold in the United States. The USP verified symbol is awarded to supplements that pass a verification process including purity, lack of harmful contaminants, and made under good manufacturing processes.

National Center for Complementary and Alternative Medicine (NCCAM)
http://www.nccam.nih.gov
PO Box 7923
Gaithersburg, MD 20898
(888) 644-6226

The Federal Government's lead agency for scientific research on the diverse medical and health care systems, practices, and products that are not generally considered part of conventional medicine.

Stress Reduction

About.com
http://stress.about.com
Information about mindfulness-based stress reduction, including a definition from About.com.

The Mayo Clinic
http://www.mayoclinic.com/health/meditation/HQ01070
Meditation tips.

A Stress Reduction Basics Guide
http://www.stressreductionbasics.com

Resources on Insurance Coverage

Center for Medicare and Medicaid Services
http://www.cms.hhs.gov

Health Resources and Services Administration (HRSA)
http://ask.hrsa.gov/pc
Federally funded healthcare centers with fees related to income plus a listing of low-cost insurance services by geographic area.

U.S. Department of Health and Human Services
http://ask.hrsa.gov/pc
Parklawn Building
5600 Fishers Lane
Rockville, MD 20857

Social Security Administration, SSA
http://www.ssa.gov
Information about retirement and disability benefits.

Health Insurance Association of America
http://www.ehealthinsurance.com
Consumer information on purchasing individual health care plans.

Coverage for Systemic Medications

Information, including generic name, brand name, and
    manufacturer.
For each therapy, patient assistance with prescription drug costs
    may be available. Search on each site for "Patient Assistance"
    for more information.

Cyclosporine (Neoral, Sandimmune; Novartis)
http://www.novartis.com

Acitretin (Soriatane; Stiefel)
http://www.soriatane.com

Infliximab (Remicade; Centocor)
http://www.remicade.com

Etanercept (Enbrel; Amgen)
http://www.enbrel.com

Alefacept (Amevive, Astellis)
http://www.amevive.com

Adalimumab (Humira; Abbott)
http://www.humira.com

Ustekinumab (Stelara; Centocor Ortho Biotech)
http://www.stelarainfo.com

Medications During Pregnancy and Breastfeeding

Pregnancy information from the FDA
http://www.4woman.gov/faq/pregmed.htm

WebMD
http://women.webmd.com/pregnancy-taking-medicine

About.com
*http://pregnancy.about.com/od/medicationinpreg/Medication_in_Preg-
nancy.htm*

Centers for Disease Control
http://www.cdc.gov/ncbddd/meds

For Children and Teens

Sleep-away summer camps for children with skin diseases. Every effort is made to offer these camps without fee to children and their families.

Camp Discovery
http://www.campdiscovery.com
A nonprofit summer camp for children and teens with skin disease. Sessions vary by age group, and there are various locations across the United States.

Camp Wonder
http://csdf.org/camp-wonder.html
A nonprofit summer camp located at Camp Arroyo, Livermore, CA.

Community Resources

Scratch That Darn Itch gives an insight into the life of someone with psoriasis.
http://stdarni.blogspot.com

Skin disease, skin conditions, and skin findings in the movies and media
http://www.skinema.com

Blog about psoriasis treatment
http://www.mypsoriasistreatment.com/blog

Project Runway
Tim Gunn, host of Project Runway, launches Fashion Therapy for Psoriasis.
Tim Gunn, whose sister suffers from psoriasis, has become a spokesperson for psoriasis treatment. He featured a fashion show in September 2009 featuring models with moderate to severe psoriasis on "Tim Gunn's Guide to Style."
http://www.addresspsoriasis.com

Glossary

Acitretin: Vitamin A derivative taken by mouth usually used to treat moderate to severe psoriasis. Sold under the trade name Soriatane.

Active ingredient: The ingredient in a topical or oral medicine that is known or expected to have a therapeutic effect.

Acute: Refers to immediate or short-term changes, usually within hours or days.

Adalimumab: A biologic therapy that works by inhibiting TNF-α. It is currently being used and under study for the treatment of moderate to severe psoriasis. Sold under the trade name Humira.

Adverse event: An unwanted change or effect caused, or thought to be caused, by a medication. Also known as a side effect.

Alefacept: A biologic therapy that works by inhibiting and eliminating T cells. It is usually used to treat moderate to severe psoriasis. Sold under the trade name Amevive.

Alternative therapy: Also called complementary therapy. An umbrella term for nonprescription medications, such as herbs and supplements, and nontraditional therapies such as acupuncture, massage, or stress reduction.

Anthralin: A derivative of tar that is used to treat psoriasis. It decreases skin inflammation but can stain skin and clothing.

Arthritis mutilans: Joint inflammation (arthritis) that causes permanent and sometimes mutilating joint changes.

Atrophy: Thinning of the skin that can be an unwanted side effect of topical steroid use. Atrophy decreases the thickness and strength of the affected skin.

Atypical presentation: A situation in which a disease arises and appears different than normal (in a different place or with a different appearance, for example), usually necessitating further tests for an accurate diagnosis.

Auspitz's sign: A skin phenomenon, often seen in psoriasis, where pinpoint spots of blood appear when a scale is lifted off the skin.

B cell: A type of white blood cell in the blood and bone marrow that makes antibodies.

Basal cell carcinoma (BCC): The most common form of skin cancer. BCC often appears as a small, shiny, raised bump on sun-exposed skin.

Base: The type of substance that a topical medicine may be formulated in (an ointment, cream, lotion, or foam).

Bath PUVA: A type of PUVA therapy where psoralen is washed over the skin in a bath, rather than taken by mouth, before UVA therapy is given.

Biologic therapy: Medical therapies that are derived from a biologic source rather than being synthesized from a chemical source.

Body surface area (BSA): The area of skin on a person, measured in square feet or square meters. Usually used as a percentage to describe the proportion of the body's skin that is affected or covered.

Calcipotriene (calcipotriol): A topically applied vitamin D derivative used to treat psoriasis. Sold under the trade name Dovonex.

Calcitriol: A topically applied vitamin D derivative used to treat psoriasis. Sold under the trade name Vectical.

Cell: The basic structural and functional unit in the human body; the building blocks of each organ and tissue.

Chromosome: A molecule of DNA found in the nucleus of every cell, chromosomes contain the cell's genetic information. Humans normally have 46 chromosomes.

Climatotherapy: Treatment of psoriasis by going to a climate that is likely to improve psoriasis due to the sunlight exposure and sometimes humidity.

Clinical diagnosis: Diagnosis based on clinical information, such as appearance and history, as opposed to being based on laboratory tests.

Clinical trial: A formally designed, officially reviewed scientific study of diagnosis, treatment, intervention, or prevention of a particular disease.

Combination therapy: Combining two or more treatments to improve effectiveness and in some cases to minimize side effects.

Complementary therapy: An umbrella term, sometimes used interchangeably with "alternative therapy," that describes nonprescription medicines, supplements, and disease therapies.

Complication: A problem that occurs after using a medication or therapy. Also known as a side effect.

Compounding: Mixing two or more different medications into a topical cream or ointment.

Corticosteroid: An umbrella term for different steroid compounds. Sometimes called steroids. These may be topical or oral.

Cream: An emulsion (mixture) of oil and water for the skin that is used to impart moisture. A cream is usually thicker than a lotion.

Crohn's disease: A chronic illness that causes irritation in the digestive tract. It occurs most commonly in the ileum (lower small intestine) or in the colon (large intestine). Along with ulcerative colitis, it is a form of inflammatory bowel disease.

Crude coal tar: Under very high temperatures, coal can be destructively distilled to crude coal tar. When applied to skin, coal tar has antibacterial, anti-itching, and photosensitizing properties.

Cyclosporine: A drug derived from a fungus that inhibits the body's immune responses. It is a common drug for patients with organ transplants and is also used in many autoimmune diseases. Sold under the trade names Sandimmune and Neoral.

Dermatologist: A physician specializing in the diagnosis and treatment of skin disease.

Dermatopathologist: A physician specializing in diagnosing skin disease by its appearance under the microscope.

Dermis: The layer of skin just underneath the epidermis that contains the skin's nerve endings, blood vessels, hair follicles, sweat glands, and immune cells.

Distal arthritis: Distal means far, so distal arthritis refers to arthritis at the ends of the limbs, like the hands and feet.

Efalizumab: A biologic therapy used to treat moderate to severe psoriasis by inhibiting T cells. Previously sold under the trade name Raptiva.

Eligibility criteria: In a clinical trial, the criteria that a patient needs to meet in order to participate. Examples include

being over age 18 or not planning to become pregnant during the study.

Epidermis: The outermost layer of skin. It is the nonvascular (without blood vessels) layer that covers and protects the dermis.

Erythema: A medical term referring to redness of the skin due to blood vessel dilation.

Erythroderma: Full-body redness of the skin due to any cause, including psoriasis.

Erythrodermic psoriasis: Full-body redness caused by psoriasis.

Etanercept: A biologic therapy that works by inhibiting TNF-α; currently usually used to treat moderate to severe psoriasis. Sold under the trade name Enbrel.

Excimer laser: A laser used by dermatologists that works at 311 nm wavelength, similar to the wavelength of UVB. It has been effective for treating psoriasis in local areas and is given in a dermatologist's office.

Foam: An inert base or vehicle made of alcohol and/or water in which an active ingredient such as a topical steroid can be mixed. A foam may appear similar in consistency to hair mousse but is used on the skin.

Food and Drug Administration (FDA): The federal organization dedicated to protecting the safety of the food and drug supply for the United States.

Gastroenterologist: A physician who specializes in diseases of the digestive tract, gall bladder, and liver.

Gene: The segment of DNA on a chromosome that contains the information necessary to make a protein. A gene is the unit of biologic inheritance.

Geographic tongue: A map-like appearance of the tongue. This results from irregular, denuded patches on its surface. It is not painful and can be found in healthy people.

Goeckerman regimen: A treatment regimen combining topical tar and light therapy, usually performed at designated psoriasis treatment centers.

Guttate psoriasis: Psoriasis that appears as little drops scattered all over the skin (instead of fewer large plaques), sometimes associated with an infection.

Heliotherapy: Treatment of psoriasis by going to a climate that is likely to improve psoriasis due to sunlight exposure.

Human leukocyte antigen (HLA) system: Proteins located on the surface of white blood cells that play an important role in our body's immune response to foreign substances.

Hyperkeratinization: Skin thickened in the outermost layer, caused by the over activity of keratinocytes in psoriasis.

Immune system: The immune system is a collection of cells and proteins that works to protect the body from potentially harmful or infectious microorganisms such as bacteria, viruses, and fungi. The immune system plays a role in the control of cancer and other diseases, but can also cause autoimmune diseases, allergies, and rejection of transplanted organs.

Immunomodulator: A medication that modifies how the immune system functions or responds.

Immunosuppressant: Anything that inhibits or weakens the immune system. Immunosuppressants can be drugs, such as prednisone and cyclosporine, or diseases, such as cancer or HIV.

Immunosuppression: Suppression of the natural immune response because immune system defenses have been suppressed, damaged, or weakened.

Indication: A symptom, like itching, or condition, like psoriasis, that can be treated through the use of a specific medical treatment or procedure.

Induration: A medical term for thickening of the skin, as sometimes seen in psoriasis.

Infliximab: A biologic antibody therapy that works by inhibiting TNF-α, approved for the treatment of psoriasis, psoriatic arthritis, and other diseases. Sold as Remicade.

Informed consent: A document that outlines a person's participation in a clinical trial. Each participant in a clinical trial in the United States must sign a consent form that explains the purpose of the trial, the results expected, how the trial works, potential risks, and a list of other treatments that are available.

Institutional Review Board (IRB): Reviews research studies that involve human participants. They ensure the ethical and safe treatment of study participants.

Intertriginous psoriasis: Psoriasis that affects intertriginous areas such as the armpits or the groin. This type of psoriasis can appear different than other types of psoriasis and may be treated differently.

Intravenous: Medication or fluid given by injection or infusion into a vein.

Inverse psoriasis: Psoriasis that affects skin folds, intertriginous areas, and/or genitals.

Iritis: Inflammation of the eye, sometimes as the result of an autoimmune disease. Also called anterior uveitis.

Keratinocyte: A skin cell of the epidermis that makes keratin, a protein that gives strength to skin, hair, and nails.

Keratolytic: A compound that helps remove dead skin cells from the epidermis and breaks down keratin in scale. One example is the group of alpha hydroxy acids.

Koebner phenomenon: This phenomenon, seen in psoriasis and other skin diseases, occurs when skin trauma initiates new lesions in previously healthy skin. Also referred to as Koebnerization.

Laser: An acronym for Light Amplification by Stimulated Emission of Radiation. A laser is a medical instrument that produces a powerful beam of light. It can produce intense heat or cool vaporization when focused at close range and is often used in medicine.

Latent tuberculosis: Tuberculosis (or TB) is an infectious disease caused by a type of bacteria. The most common target of the disease is the lungs. In some people, the disease may remain quiet without symptoms, but the bacterium is present. This state is referred to as latent TB and can reactivate if a person starts taking an immunosuppressive therapy.

Lipids: Cholesterol and other fats found in the bloodstream, such as triglycerides.

Liquor carbonis detergens (LCD): Crude coal can be refined with alcohol extraction to yield liquor carbonis detergens (LCD). This type of tar therapy works like other tar types to decrease skin inflammation.

Liver biopsy: The removal of a small piece of tissue from the liver using a special needle. The tissue is then examined under a microscope to look for the presence of inflammation or liver damage.

Local effects: Effects of a medication, either beneficial or unwanted, that appear only at the site of administration. For example, a topical corticosteroid could treat psoriasis locally, or could cause local skin thinning.

Lotion: A water-based, or water- and alcohol-based, topical medication used to treat the skin, sometimes called a "solution."

Medical dermatology: The branch of dermatology that treats medical diseases of the skin, such as psoriasis, that may need systemic drug therapy, or skin changes that arise from systemic diseases.

Medicare: The primary health insurance program for people over the age of 65 and those with certain disabilities. Medicare provides for acute hospital care, physician services, short stays in nursing facilities, and short-term home care for a medical problem. Coverage is restricted to medical care, to prescription drugs under certain limits, though not custodial care at home or in a nursing home. It was established by Congress in 1935.

Melanocyte: The skin cells that produce melanin (the primary pigment that gives skin its color) and are found in the basal layer of the epidermis.

Methotrexate: A cytotoxic (cell-killing) immunosuppressive drug that is used in high doses for the treatment of cancer and in lower doses for autoimmune disorders.

Mucous membranes: The linings of the mouth, nose, vagina, and urethra (inside of the penis). These moist skin areas secrete mucous to keep the surfaces moist.

Narrow-band UVB: Narrow-band UVB refers to a specific wavelength of UV radiation (311 to 313 nm). This range has proven the most beneficial component of natural sunlight for psoriasis.

National Institutes of Health (NIH): The National Institutes of Health is the primary center for medical research in the United States, as well as one of the world's leading research centers. It is the agency within the Department of Health and Human Services responsible for most of its medical research programs and related functions, including the National Library of Medicine.

National Psoriasis Foundation: The largest not-for-profit national organization dedicated to helping people with psoriasis.

Neutrophil: The most common type of white blood cell in the bloodstream, it helps defend against bacterial infections. When these cells accumulate in large areas, pus is formed.

NIH: See *National Institutes of Health.*

Nonsteroidal anti-inflammatories (NSAIDs): Aspirin, ibuprofen (the active ingredient in Motrin or Advil), indomethacin, and some other painkillers have both anti-inflammatory and anti-pain properties. These medications are distinct from steroid-based anti-inflammatories such as prednisone and dexamethasone, and distinct from acetaminophen (Tylenol).

Nutritional supplement: As defined by the FDA, a nutritional supplement is a product intended to supplement the diet that contains one or more of the following dietary ingredients: a vitamin, a mineral, an herb or other botanical, an amino acid, or a dietary substance to supplement the diet by increasing the total daily intake.

Occlusion: Covering, for example, with cotton (cotton socks or gloves), plastic wrap, or tape.

Off-label prescribing: The common and accepted practice of using a prescription medication for a purpose other than the one for which it was approved.

Oil spot: A description of the appearance of small spots (1 to 4 mm) on the nail in psoriasis. These occur when the nail separates from the skin below because of psoriasis in the nail bed.

Ointment: A topical formulation that mixes an active ingredient into a base of solely petrolatum (Vaseline) without any water content. Medications can be mixed into ointments for topical use. Among topical formulas, ointments tend to be the most effective.

Oligoarthritis: Inflammation of a few (oligo-) joints (-arthritis).

Onycholysis: A medical term for nail splitting and crumbling, whether from psoriasis or another cause such as a fungus.

Orthopedist: A surgeon concerned with the diagnosis, care, and treatment of musculoskeletal disorders. (Also known as orthopedic surgeon.)

Over-the-counter (OTC): Products (medications, creams, vitamins, supplements, etc.) available at the drugstore. These medications can be effective but are not usually covered by medical insurance.

Paint PUVA: A special type of PUVA where psoralen is "painted" directly onto the skin before exposure to UVA light in the same area.

Palmar-plantar psoriasis: Psoriasis on the hands and feet. This psoriasis may appear different from other types. (Also called palmoplantar psoriasis.)

PASI Score: A specialized way to measure changes in psoriasis severity used in research studies. It incorporates psoriasis area and psoriasis activity (redness, thickness, and scale). PASI 75 indicates a 75% improvement in the PASI score, often used to track improvement in studies of new medications; PASI 50 is a 50% improvement in the PASI score.

Pathology report: The formal report of a physician after looking at a skin sample under the microscope. This report is part of a patient's medical record.

Petrolatum: A semi-solid mixture of hydrocarbons that is inert and free of water molecules. Vaseline and Aquaphor are commonly used brands of petrolatum. It can be used alone as an ointment or mixed in with other medications.

Photoaging: The naturally occurring aging process that progresses during a lifetime of sun exposure.

Phototherapy: The use of light, whether from the sun or special light sources, to treat skin disease.

Pimecrolimus: A topical immunomodulator that can be used for psoriasis, especially on genitals and skin folds. Sold under the trade name Elidel.

Plaque: In psoriasis, an area of skin affected by the disease.

Plaque psoriasis: The most common form of psoriasis, also called psoriasis vulgaris.

Polyarthritis: A medical term referring to arthritis in many (poly-) joints (-arthritis).

Post-inflammatory changes: Darker or lighter areas of skin that develop after a skin injury, such as psoriasis or an ordinary scrape, resolves.

Potency: A way to describe the strength of a medication. It may be measured by the concentration or amount used, or measured, relative to a standard (hydrocortisone for topical steroids).

PPD, or "Purified Protein Derivative," Test: A skin test for previous exposure to tuberculosis. Certain tuberculosis proteins are injected under the skin, and after a few days the skin is checked to see if the body mounts a response (shown as a raised, red wheal). The PPD test can be positive in people who have had a tuberculosis vaccine as a child (given in some foreign countries) or exposure in the past. People with positive tests usually need a chest x-ray to check for any tuberculosis in the lungs.

Preauthorization: Pretreatment clearance from an insurance company to use a particular therapy. The process usually involves a physician corresponding with an insurance company on a patient's behalf.

Prednisone: A type of cortisone (a so-called "stress hormone" naturally made by the body) that can be taken by mouth.

Prescription drug: A drug available only by the prescription of a physician. These drugs have been formally tested and are regulated by the FDA.

Ps, Pso: Abbreviation used for psoriasis.

PsA, PsoA: Abbreviation used for psoriatic arthritis.

Psoralen: A medicine that, when taken by mouth or put onto the skin, increases the skin's sensitivity to UVA light. In combination with UVA light, it is called PUVA and is used to treat psoriasis and other skin diseases.

Psoriasis Area Severity Index (PASI): A measurement that combines BSA with a rating of the severity of scaling, thickness, and redness in a particular area. A PASI score approximates with a number the severity of psoriasis.

Psoriasis vulgaris: The most common form of psoriasis, it usually appears as scaly, red plaques on the elbows, knees, and scalp.

Psoriatic arthritis: A term for the several types of arthritis that can develop in people with psoriasis. It is distinct from other common types of arthritis and may need to be treated differently.

Pulse treatment: The planned use of a very strong or very high-dose medication for a short period of time.

Punch biopsy: A biopsy that uses a small, specially designed punching tool shaped like a miniature "cookie cutter." This punch is usually deeper than a shave and lets the examining physician see farther down into the skin.

Pustular psoriasis: A type of psoriasis where sterile (uninfected) pustules appear on the skin.

PUVA: The use of psoralen medication, by mouth or on the skin, combined with UVA light to treat psoriasis.

Rebound: In psoriasis, a rapid worsening of skin disease; typically the psoriasis worsens beyond its original severity after a medication is stopped.

Rheumatologist: A physician who specializes in diseases of the immune system and the joints.

Rotational therapy: Rotating different therapies over time in order to maximize benefits while minimizing side effects that might accumulate.

Sacroiliac joint: The joints between the hip bones and the spine.

Sequential therapy: Transitioning from one therapy to another to maximize certain treatment characteristics. An example would be starting with a medication that works rapidly to initiate clearing and following it with a slower-acting medication that may be safer for long-term use.

Shave biopsy: A biopsy performed with a razor by cutting off a superficial piece of the skin.

Side effect: An undesired effect of a medication.

Skin: The largest organ of the body, acting as a physically protective covering, site of the sense of touch, and a border of immune surveillance.

Skin biopsy: The surgical removal of a piece of skin (often the size of a pencil eraser) for examination under a microscope. A biopsy is often done to diagnose a skin disease.

Solution: A mixture of a medicine in water, or water with alcohol, for topical use, often on hair-bearing areas. Sometimes referred to as a "lotion."

Spondylarthropathy: Inflammation of the spine and hip joints.

Squamous cell carcinoma (SCC): The second most common skin cancer, it arises from the epidermis and resembles the squamous cells that comprise most of the upper layers of skin. This may occur anywhere on the body, including the mucous membranes, but are most common in areas exposed to the sun.

Stelara: See *Ustekinumab*.

Steroid: A large class of pharmaceutical agents that chemically resemble cholesterol. Two well-known types are glucocorticoid steroids, used to reduce inflammation, and anabolic steroids, which are often used (illegally) in athletics.

Subcutaneous: The tissue just below the surface of the skin. Some medicines are injected into this area.

Superinfection: An infection that develops following another skin problem, such as psoriasis or eczema, for example. This infection is often more persistent or more difficult to treat than an infection on previously healthy skin.

Suture: A medical term for a stitch. Some sutures may need to be removed, while others can dissolve on their own.

Synergism: When the benefits of two medications used together are even greater than what they would be if they were simply added because they complement each other in some way.

Systemic: Something that reaches or affects the entire body.

Systemic absorption: The absorption of a medication through the skin, for example, into the blood where it reaches the entire body.

Systemic effects: Effects of a medication that reach throughout the body and therefore may affect organs or systems beyond the skin or joints.

Systemic medication: A medication given, either by mouth or by injection, to reach the entire body.

Systemic steroids: Steroids that are given orally, by injection, or by vein and therefore have many different effects on the body.

Systemic therapy or treatment: Medications that are given in ways that make it likely that they will be absorbed throughout the body, and therefore have the potential to affect organs and systems other than the skin or joints.

T cell: A type of white blood cell that attacks foreign and infected cells to protect the body.

Tachyphylaxis: The phenomenon where a medication becomes less effective over a long period of use.

Taclonex: An ointment made of the combination of calcipotriene and the steroid bethamethsone for use on body psoriasis.

Tacrolimus: A topical immunomodulator, usually used for eczema, that can be effective in genital and other types of psoriasis. Also comes in an oral form used in transplantation and sometimes in psoriasis. Sold under the trade name Protopic.

Tar: A brown or black material, liquid or semisolid in consistency, derived from coal, petroleum, wood, or other organic material. Used on the skin, it has immunosuppressant qualities and has long been used to treat psoriasis.

Tazarotene: A topical vitamin A derivative developed to treat psoriasis. An oral form is in development. Sold under the trade name Tazorac.

Therapy holiday: A scheduled time without therapy, planned by a patient and his or her physician.

Topical treatment: A treatment administered on the skin to treat an infection locally.

Ultraviolet (UV) radiation: Invisible rays that are part of the energy that comes from the sun. It is made up of two types of rays: UVA and UVB.

Ustekinumab (sold as Stelara): A biologic inhibitor of the cytokines interleukin 12 and 23 that is used to treat psoriasis.

UVA: A particular wavelength of light that is used in combination with a medication called psoralen to treat psoriasis.

UVB: A particular wavelength of light that can be used alone to treat psoriasis.

Vehicle: The base or inactive product into which a medication is mixed. Examples include petrolatum, cream, and foam.

Wavelength: The length of a particular wave of light. These lengths vary in different types of light (ultraviolet vs. visible light or different types of UV light, for example) and help determine how far into the skin these waves will penetrate.

White blood cell: A specialized type of cell present in the blood that works to fight against infection.

Woronoff ring: A ring of pale-appearing skin that may be visible at the edge of a psoriasis plaque.

Index

Index

L

labetolol, 21
laser therapy, 61, 62
legs, psoriasis on, 23, 24
leprosy graecorum, 5
less common manifestations, 19–20
leukemia, 29
lichen planus, 6
licorice extract, 121
lifelong nature, of psoriasis, 25
life-threatening psoriasis, 17
light box, 61
    tanning bed vs., 98–99
light therapy, 22, 29, 94, 133
    long-term risks of, 96
    reasons for choosing, 97
    sunlight, 5, 21–22, 49, 61, 74, 94, 133,
        154–155
    types of, 95
        Goeckerman regimen, 95–96, 97–98
        Ingram regimen, 96, 97–98
liquor carbonis detergens, 74–75
lithium, 21
liver biopsy, 100, 101, 102–103
liver function, 101, 111–112
    damage, 100
    disease, 32
local effects, 71–72
lotion, 60, 73, 92
    choosing among medication formations,
        75–76
lower back, psoriatic arthritis, 43
lupus, skin forms of, 6
lymphoma, 29

M

makeup, permanent, 51
massage, 122
medical record, 13
Medicare, 65–66, 115
medicated shampoo, 76, 90
medications, 14; *See also* side effects;
        steroids
    bring list to doctor appointment, 32
    choosing among formations of, 75–76
    compounding, 84
    drug safety for children, 73
    exacerbating symptoms, 12, 20
        classes known to cause flare-ups, 21
    guttate psoriasis triggered by, 42
    immunosuppressive, 24, 30, 100
    injectable, 60, 72
        biologics, 111–112
    intravenous, 30, 60, 72

local effects, 71–72
new, 33
    clinical trials, 115–118, 136
    oral, 60, 128
        dosages and time periods, 70
    over-the-counter products, 26, 66
    during pregnancy, 101, 132, 133, 164
    prescription, 65–66
    questions for dermatologist, 68–69
    reported to worsen psoriasis, 125–126
    stopping, 129–130
    subcutaneous, risk from, 29–30
    "therapy holiday," 80
meditation, 20, 122, 163
melanocyte, 3
menopause, 153–154
metabolism, drugs affecting, 61
methotrexate, 61, 99, 100, 101, 128, 133
metoprolol, 21
milk, 49
milk thistle, 49
mites, 15
monitoring, of biologics, 111–112
Motrin. *See* ibuprofen, 37
mouth, 2
mucous membrane, 2, 19, 73
mupirocin (Bactroban), 51
musculoskeletal disorders, 14
mycophenolate mofetil, 61

N

nail dystrophy, 35
nail psoriasis, 19, 23, 44
    treatment, 65, 90–92
naproxen, 21
narrow-band UVB, 62
National Institutes of Health (NIH), 156
National Psoriasis Foundation, 15, 36, 50,
        66, 67, 161
    doctor referrals from, 70–71
    light therapy referrals from, 97
    listing of promising new trials, 116
Native Americans, 9
"natural," 122
neomycin (Neosporin), 51
Neoral. *See* cyclosporine
Neosporin. *See* neomycin
nerves, 2, 3
neutrophils, 4
NIH. *See* National Institutes of Health
nonsteroidal anti-inflammatories
        (NSAIDS), 21, 37
northern Europe, 10
nose, 2

NSAIDS. *See* nonsteroidal
anti-inflammatories
nutritional supplements, 156

O

obesity, 29
occlusion, 64, 77
off-label prescribing, 115
oil spot, 35
ointment, 92
choosing among medication formations,
75–76
oligoarthritis, 38
onycholysis, 35
ophthalmologist, 19
oral medications, 60, 128
dosages and time periods, 70
oral steroids, when suddenly stopped, 21
erythrodermic psoriasis, 43, 44
oregano oil, 49
orthopedic surgeon, 14
orthopedist, 14, 34
osteoarthritis, 28–29, 34
"wear and tear" vs. psoriatic, 37–38
OTC. *See* over-the-counter products
over-the-counter (OTC) products, 26, 66

P

paint PUVA, 92–93
palmar-plantar psoriasis, 7, 17
symptoms, 42
treatment, 42, 64, 92–93
PASI Score, 118
pathology report, 13
penis, 2; *See also* genital psoriasis
petrolatum, 51, 60, 75, 85
pharmaceuticals. *See* medications
photoaging, 74; *See also* age, of patient
phototherapy, 22
erythrodermic psoriasis from, 43
pimecrolimus (Elidel), 42, 63, 65, 82, 93
genital psoriasis, 44
pregnancy category, 133
pityriasis rosea, 6
plaque psoriasis, 9, 17
treatment, 64, 65
plaques, scaly, 5
formation of, 7–8
polyarthritis, 38
polymyxin (Polysporin), 51
Polysporin. *See* polymyxin
potency, 78–79
PPD test, 30
preauthorization, 66

prednisone, 21
pregnancy, 130–131, 153–154
medications during, 101, 132, 133, 164
prenatal diagnostic, 46
prescription drug, 65–66
refills, 130
ProGraf. *See* tacrolimus
progressive multifocal leukoencephalopathy,
108
propranolol, 21
PsA/PsoA, 36
psora leprosa, 5
psoralen, 92, 97, 133
psoriasis; *See also* diagnosis; treatment
causes of, 7–9
cure for, 18–19
famous people with, 157–158
fluctuation over time, 46–47
heartbreak of, 26
infection risk with, 126–127
less common manifestations of, 19–20
in movies, 158–159, 165
prevalence rates, 9–10
remission, 47–48
risk of other diseases with, 28–29
severe/critical, 17, 23–24, 43, 47
talking about, 148–150
types of, 37–38, 40
worldwide prevalence, 10
psoriasis vulgaris, 9, 15
common bodily locations, 16
psoriatic arthritis, 10, 19, 28
differential diagnosis, 33–34
CASPAR criteria, 34–35
x-ray, 34
therapy, 35–36
systemic, 37
types of, 37–38
"wear and tear" osteoarthritic vs.,
37–38
who gets it?, 35
Ps/Pso, 36
pulse dosing, 100, 128
punch biopsy, 30–31
pus. *See* neutrophils
pustular psoriasis, 7, 17, 23, 52–53
treatment for, 43
PUVA, bath, 97
PUVA light therapy, 22, 61, 64, 92–93
for palmar-plantar, 42
risk of skin cancer with, 29

Q

qi (vital energy), 122

Index